The Kinesiologies Handbook

The

KINESIOLOGIES

HANDBOOK

Volume 2

by

Dr Harry Howell

(DSc, PhD, Dr Ac, ND, MK, FCAS)

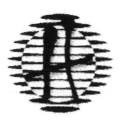

Hub House Publishing

1

Also by Harry Howell:

Health Books:

The Kinesiologies Handbook, Volume 1

The Kinesiologies Handbook, Volume 2

HER Inner Games of Sex

HIS Inner Games of Sex

How to DUMP Your Depression - & Start Living Again

Pain Relief – Made Simple

Novels:

The Swastika Connection

Dead Fall

Mouth of the Inferno

Published in the USA by Hub House Publishing

ISBN: 13:978-1499345759

ISBN-10:1499345755

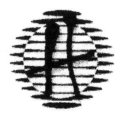

Contents

Chapter 1

Introduction to Sex Kinesiology – Female (SKF)

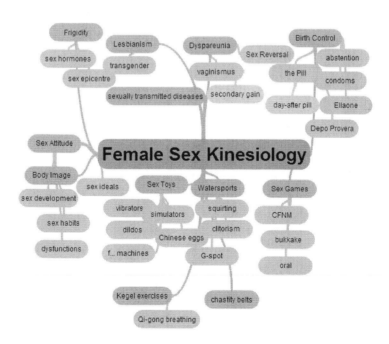

"Sexual love is undoubtedly one of the chief things in life, and the union of mental and bodily satisfaction in the enjoyment of love is one of its culminating peaks"
(SigmundFreud)

"I kissed my first girl and smoked my first cigarette on the same day. I haven't had time for tobacco since."
(Arturo Toscanini)

"Sex is God's joke on human beings." (Bette Davis)

"A man on a date wonders if he'll get lucky.
The woman already knows." (Monica Piper)

"It is not enough to conquer; one must know how to seduce." (Voltaire)

Sex and love are not the same thing. Sex can be achieved without love, and love does not necessarily involve sex. They are both influenced as much by culture as by nature, despite being one of the most powerful natural instincts. It can be practised with or without skill, for procreation or just for pleasure, with or without a partner, with the same or opposite gender, or even – *in extremis* – with a different species.

"Sex appeal is 50% what you've got and 50% what people *think* you've got," Sophia Loren once said, and maybe that sums up what this book is about. The psyche, the way we think about things, plays an enormous part in human sexual practice, yet comparatively little has been written about it – in the West, anyway.

In India, China and other parts of the Orient, they have been writing about it for thousands of years. The basic principles in Oriental sexual philosophies are

- Regulation of ejaculation
- The importance of female satisfaction
- That male orgasm, ejaculation and satisfaction are not the same things
- The arts of the sexual act (and the use of aphrodisiacs)

The Yellow Emperor, *Huang Di*, who is considered to be the father of Chinese Medicine, is the author of the *Nei Jing*. It is the oldest known treatise on sexual health. The opinions in the Nei Jing were accepted equally by the two contradictory philosophical schools – the Confucianists and the Taoists. Their conviction was that sexual intercourse elevated man above the terrestrial plane, and that at the moment of orgasm he and Yin transcended into an even wider union with the Cosmos, and that in order to assure the frequency of this euphoric state, man should learn as much as possible about the art of the techniques of lovemaking.

With so much importance, both social and political, given to the sex act, it was not surprising that this aspect of court life was not confined only to the royal bedchamber. The palace, or indeed courts with many palaces, was the setting for orgies and sex carnivals, excesses and strange practices, which could be justified by their contribution to the total Yin-Yang harmony generated for the benefit of the entire community.

"The big difference between sex for money and sex for free is that sex for money costs less," said Brendan Francis. Which raises the question of the vast sex industry, ranging from modelling clothes to selling cars on TV, to prostitution and hard-core pornography. The enormity of the subject makes it impossible to cram everything into one book, but we'll try and deal with some of the sex problems here and leave the rest for another time.

Female Frigidity

"There are no frigid women, only inept men."
(Alfred Kinsey)

Although there are some similarities between this and some male sexual dysfunctions, most of the causes of frigidity within women are psychogenic.

It is a condition in which women are generally unresponsive to sexual stimulation, and who generally attain little or no erotic pleasure. It is not to be confused with sexual anaesthesia, in which a female may actually enjoy sexual contact with a male although unable to actually enjoy a sensation of touch.

In physiological terms, the normal female response to stimulation would be vaginal lubrication, swelling and colouration of the vaginal walls, engorgement of the clitoris, and formation of the orgasmic platform.

With <u>General Sexual Dysfunction</u> (a long-winded term generally preferred to frigidity) these physical responses are lacking, although it is possible for an orgasm to be experienced despite these impairments.

- *Primary* frigidity refers to a female who has never had intercourse, and has never experienced erotic pleasure with any partner at any time.
- *Secondary* frigidity refers to one who has had intercourse or erotic pleasure at some time.
- *Tertiary* frigidity applies to a female who is sexually unresponsive to her husband or normal partner but can enjoy sex with another partner.

In Primary cases, there is often a case of repressive upbringing, either by strict parents or for orthodox religious reasons. Occasionally, it is as the result of a frightening childhood experience, e.g. child molesting, witnessing something unpleasant (mother having sex with stranger, exposure of penis, perhaps in a threatening way, by a stranger), or even a male sibling, uncle or father who has behaved in some sexual manner towards her. It may also be the result of a hysteric personality disorder.

Secondary cases, much more common and diverse in causative factors, can often be traced back to a childbirth (not necessarily the first), tiredness or depression, living in crowded conditions, may be concerned about becoming pregnant, menstrual irregularity or pain (*dysmennorhoea*), or feelings of resentment towards husband or partner, to name just a few.

Factors which reduce erotic interest for a female include:

- lack of sexual interest in partner
- inadequate stimulation
- poor communication with partner
- anxiety or acute tension
- shame/guilt due to restrictive upbringing or religious beliefs
- fear of losing control
- fear of rejection through failure to satisfy partner
- fear of pregnancy
- fear of partner (perhaps aggressive, sadistic, brutal, heavy drinker, etc.)
- will permit sex only out of marital duty

As a result of any of these characteristics, the female protects herself by erecting a defensive barrier. The job of therapy is to penetrate the barrier and reach the areas of sensitivity beneath.

Sexual attraction, the ability to have orgasms, and many other sexual characteristics, are essentially a question of culture. Sudanese, Ethiopian, and many other African countries have a custom of female circumcision – usually illegal but nevertheless still practised – which is a device to prevent a woman from having an orgasm. The recognised role of such women is to bear children.

In our own culture, within the last few years, sex has been discussed more openly than at any time within the last century. Improved methods of contraception have meant that many more women are now predisposed to have sex for its own sake, and they feel – quite rightly – that they are entitled to be able to enjoy it.

But there are still many other factors that can prevent a female from enjoying sex. She may be physically attracted to a partner but regard him as stupid, coarse, or unintelligent. She may wish to reward him on some occasions and punish him on others. Sex, in fact, can often be used as a bargaining factor within a relationship – even a marital one.

There is also the question of leading and dominance. Some females prefer to be led, others to lead. She may have contempt for a partner lacking expertise, or who is selfish sexually. Or she may wish to totally dominate a man or, conversely, be totally dominated.

If a partner is contrary to any of these deeply felt desires, the result may be a total disinterest in sex or a particular partner. Some women prefer 'gentle' lovers, others prefer their partner to be more forceful, or manly. Some prefer younger men, others the older type.

Some women even set out to be 'vengeful' on all men in return for some historical event causing them unhappiness. The role of the father may be important here, if one is looking for historical causes.

Some women are able to appear passionate and willing simply in order to enable their partner to ejaculate quickly – even before penetration, perhaps – and thus bring a quick end to the ordeal.

Unlike men, who are rarely affected sexually through hormone imbalance, this is somewhat more likely with females, and there are a number of cases where an increase in *testosterone* has a definite effect.

The principal female sex hormones are androgen and oestrogen, and it has been discovered that females seem to lose all sexual interest when the source of androgen production is removed by surgery. When given testosterone, however, they become highly sexually aroused. Because it is essentially a male sex hormone, and only produced in females in small quantities, care has to be taken to avoid masculinising side-effects, e.g. hirsutism (excess body or facial hair).

Physical, medical and organic causes for lowering sexual desire within females includes the following:

- infections
- any chronic painful illness
- renal, pulmonary and cardiac diseases
- malignancies
- advanced stages of diabetes
- dyspareunia
- vaginismus
- ovarian tumours and cysts
- anal fissures
- haemorrhoids
- vaginal polyps
- prolapsed uterus
- any inflammation of the pelvis

With post-partum secondary frigidity, a good clue is the post-natal examination, usually about 6 weeks after birth. If female indicates to her partner that she wants to wait until after the examination before renewing intercourse it is often the case that general sexual dysfunction is taking place.

Hypoactive or Sexual Aversion?

Hypoactive sexual desire disorder is regarded as the most common sexual problem for women. Criteria necessary for this diagnosis include persistently deficient or absent sexual fantasies and/or desire for sexual activity.

This must be considered in cases where the lack of sexual interest causes marked distress or interpersonal difficulty. The first enquiry here must be to eliminate any organic problems as a possible cause.

The most likely cause is a hormone deficiency, especially testosterone, or DHEA. The next one to test for (kinesiologically) is serotonin.

Sexual aversion disorder is where a female avoids any sexual contact, usually of a genital nature, although in rare kisses this can include kissing or even touching.

The effect, when confronted with a sexual opportunity is usually anxiety, fear or disgust. This condition generally affects females who have been through some type of sexual crisis, such as rape, gang rape, forced sex, or sex with a family member. This disorder is also very common in religious as some faiths have very strict rules about sexual activity.

Dryness

Lack of lubrication can also be a cause of female frigidity. This is a condition often seen in young women, and in those cases is nearly always caused as a side effect of birth control pills or shots.

Another cause can be diabetes, especially in long-standing cases. This would also cause lack of blood to the sex organs, which could result in fungal or bacterial infections of the nether regions.

Radiation treatments can also cause lack of lubrication. This may be due to treatment for breast lumps or cancer. The drug Tamoxifen can also cause dryness. Vitamin E suppositories can be helpful in these cases.

Dryness of the vagina is also seen in breast-feeding mothers, due to a high elevation of prolactin, which can also cause a lack of interest in sex.

So, eliminating all these variables is important. Testing and treating the Bartholin glands, as described in Dyspareunia is one approach. When everything fails, synthetic lubrication can be considered. Only water-soluble lubricants should be used as they don't usually create new problems. Silicon lubricants are also usually problem-free. But avoid all petroleum-based lubricants, such as Vaseline. They're sticky, and can harbour bacteria.

QUESTIONNAIRE

Sexual Attitudes

1. Do you believe you have a basic human right to enjoy sex?
2. Is the main purpose of sex to produce children, or for pleasure?
3. Do you find some sexual practices disgusting?
4. Are you willing to try anything at least once?
5. Do you believe that a male should dominate sexually?
6. Do you believe it is a woman's duty to please her partner sexually?
7. Do you feel sexually attracted towards your partner?
8. Do you hold any religious convictions regarding sex?

Outline of Dysfunctions

1. Under what circumstances have you experienced an orgasm, if ever?
2. Has your sexual relationship with present partner been happy? If not, at what point did it become unsatisfactory?

3. How long have you had this relationship?

4. What previous relationships have you had?

5. Did you experience sexual satisfaction or not?

6. Has your partner tried means other than intercourse to bring sexual pleasure to you? Describe.

7. Describe your first sexual experience within the present relationship.

8. Are the non-sexual areas of your relationship satisfactory? Describe.

9. Have you participated in any extra-marital activities within this relationship? If so, have they been sexually satisfying?

10. If so, is your partner aware of them?

11. To your knowledge, has your partner indulged in any extra-marital activities?

12. Has your partner experienced any erectile or ejaculatory difficulty?

13. Have you, at any time, experienced sexual happiness? Describe.

Sexual Development

1. At what age did you first experience a genital feeling of pleasure?

2. At what age did you first experiment with masturbation?

3. How did you first learn about masturbation?

4. How frequently did you pursue masturbation?
5. Have you masturbated during the present relationship (a) with partner's knowledge? (b) without partner's knowledge?
6. Do you experience orgasm (a) through masturbation (b) through intercourse (c) not at all?
7. Do you enjoy being touched by partner?
8. Was there ever a time when you did enjoy being touched by partner?
9. What prevents your enjoyment of it now?
10. What was your principal attraction to your partner?
11. Is that attraction still there today?
12. Have you ever been asked to perform a sexual act you regard as disgusting?
13. Have you ever been forced to perform a sexual act you find disgusting?
14. How frequently did you have intercourse in the early part of this present relationship?
15. Was that frequency satisfactory to you?
16. What frequency might you have preferred, given the choice?

Medical

1. Have you ever had any surgery? Describe.
2. Have you ever had any serious illness?

3. Have you ever been treated for depression? If so, what treatment was prescribed? Note any of the following medications: methadone, morphine, demerol, codeine, heroin (all have a depressive action on the Central Nervous System)

Sexual Behaviour

1. Does lovemaking usually lead to intercourse?
2. Where does sex usually take place?
3. At what time of day?
4. Who has the greatest influence on sex, you or your partner?
5. What turns you on most?
6. What turns you off most?
7. Are you able to discuss sex openly with partner?
8. Does your partner have any sexual habits you dislike?
9. Does your partner stimulate you adequately?
10. Do you ever fear losing control of yourself during sex?
11. Are you concerned about failing to satisfy your partner?
12. Do you ever worry about becoming pregnant? Frequently?
13. Does your partner frighten you sometimes?

14. How do you feel about touching partner's genitals?
15. How do you feel about partner touching your genitals?
16. Do you place any limitations on partner (i.e. Not to touch certain parts)?
17. Do you ever fake an orgasm to please partner? Frequently?

Body Image

1. What do you think of your hair? Style, texture, colour?
2. How about your eyes?
3. Nose. Are you satisfied with it?
4. Would you like it changed in any way?
5. How about your mouth? Are you satisfied with it?
6. Voice. How do you feel about your voice?
7. What about your arms?
8. How about your hands?
9. Your overall figure. What do you think about it? Height, weight, etc.
10. How about your breasts? Are they too big, too small, too saggy?
11. And the nipples. How do you feel about them?
12. Are your breasts and nipples sensitive to touch?

13. How about your stomach? How do you feel about your stomach?

14. And how about your hips?

15. Genitals. How do you feel about your genitals?

16. How about your pubic hair? Are you conscious of it?

17. Do you feel that your vagina is too small? Too tight? Too loose?

18. How about your clitoris? Is it sensitive to touch?

19. Do you try to avoid exposing your genitals to anyone? To partner?

20. What about your buttocks? Satisfied?

21. Thighs. How do you feel about your thighs?

22. Legs?

23. Feet? Satisfied with your feet? And your toes?

24. How about your personality? How do you feel about that?

25. How do you feel about your partner's body?

Ideal

1. Can you describe how you think a sexual encounter should be?

2. Have you ever experienced anything like that?

3. Do you think it is possible to achieve the ideal?

4. What things are you good at (sexually)?

5. What things are you not good at (sexually)?

*　　　*　　　*

Because women often use sex as a weapon – they frequently find it's the only weapon they have – there is sometimes a tendency to look negatively at the whole purpose of sex. They are threatened and coerced sexually during their childhood, and underlying sexual tensions lead them to associate sex with fear.

This, together with the fact that sex has virtually been controlled by men, means that females often feel that they are little more than 'sexual objects' in the eyes of men, to be exploited and used, and very often just dumped when that usefulness is over.

It is often considered all right for men to have a little sex on the side, a night out at a strip show, a stag night, and so on. Society is changing in its attitudes towards sex but only slowly, and for some women not at all.

So male therapists, in particular, need to understand and accept that sex in the minds of many, if not most, females is not the same as in the eyes of men.

While boys in adolescence often get encouragement from father to go out and get some experience, many adolescent girls get strict warnings from mother. This might be particularly severe in cases where mother herself has been sexually suppressed and victimised.

These childhood warnings can become deeply imprinted and prevent normal sexual release. Masturbation might have been regarded as something dirty, and even the naked body itself not to be scarcely looked at, even by its owner. So one often finds, in therapy, that there is a reluctance to talk about body images, masturbation, and other similar topics of a very personal nature.

Inhibitions of feeling can often be quickly detected by inhibitions of breathing, so we can use deep breathing to help people get down to deep feelings. And increased awareness of body is important.

Client should be urged to start taking more note of her body, perhaps standing in front of a full-length mirror and carefully observing every part of herself, gently touching each part to see how much sensitivity exists there.

The genitals can best be examined by using a hand-held mirror, and particular attention should be paid to the clitoris. Clients need to start developing sensitivity to touch, which may be something she has carefully avoided. Touching herself, lightly at first, and then sensually, can gradually be developed until it leads to self-stimulation. Some clients may need advice on how to do this. Many books are available on the subject .

Case Study 1

Alison C, aged 23:

"Since the age of about twelve I seem to have attracted the sexual attention of men and boys alike. By male standards, I appear to be 'pretty' and, as it has often been said, 'have all the right things in the right places and in the right proportions'. Even at school, which was all girls, I never seemed to want to get involved in any of the sexual practices I saw going on in the showers and dormitory at night. Some of the girls used to poke fun at me and call me silly prudish names, but if anything that only had the effect of making me more determined not to get drawn into their games. After I left school, I did go out a few times with a lad who worked near where I live. One time he took me to the pictures and insisted on sitting in the back row. He kissed me a few times, which I didn't resist although it didn't do anything for me. He tried to feel my breasts but I just kept pushing his hand away. Then he took hold of my hand and before I realised what he was doing had placed it on his penis, which I could feel was hard.

Fortunately, it was still in his trousers, and I quickly pulled my hand away and resisted any further attempts by him to do the same again. Since that date, I've had several attempts by men to have some sort of sex with me, but I have never had the slightest interest. I can also say that I have never attempted masturbation simply because it just hasn't held any interest for me."

When Alison first came to me I had no idea about an underlying cause for her condition. But an important factor was *she felt that she was abnormal.* Despite her insistence that she had never experienced sexual stimulation, the very fact that she had come to me of her own free will was an indication that was unhappy about herself because, despite her frigidity, she still felt that she liked being in male company and wanted a 'normal' relationship.

After our first session I said I wanted to try hypnosis with her. Not surprisingly, her first reaction was to resist. I did finally manage to get her consent after I explained that hypnosis was only a deep relaxation, that she would be aware of being said, and she could bring herself out of it at anytime if she so wanted.

The first hypnotic session was nothing more than introducing her to a deep relaxation and I didn't attempt any exploration into her past. At the next session I suggested it might be a good idea to try and trace back into the past and she agreed without hesitation. I took her into a medium-deep trance and asked her to just slide back into a free-form mode and talk about anything related to the 'problem' of her apparent lack of interest in sex.

This is a direct excerpt from that second session:

"I can see myself lying on top of a bed. I'm dressed in a green skirt and white blouse. My eyes are closed. I think I'm sleeping. Now I'm being drawn in … as if I'm going inside myself. Everything is suddenly dark and quiet. In the distance is a tiny speck of light, growing quickly … with a rush, as if I'm on a train going through a tunnel and the light is coming closer and closer … Now everything's changed … I'm looking down into a room … Mrs P. [Alison's teacher] is there, standing in a corner with a dunce's hat on … she has no clothes on … now I'm in the room with her, sitting on the floor in the corner … Mrs P. is bending down over me, I try to cover my eyes, she has a large fat belly and a huge mat of brown hair going from her navel down to her … pussy. She's pulling my arm away from her face, making me look at her. Her other hand is parting the hair from her ... I don't want to look but she's holding my eyes open ... I'm starting to lick the lower part of her body ... I'm licking her breasts now ... I can see her dark hair coming from her armpits and worms wriggling out of it ... I'm vomiting all over her now and she's slapping my face and screaming at me ... I'm going to the toilet all over the floor, I scream, I cry ... I'm spraying everywhere with shit and piss, over Mrs P., over myself ... the scene is changing very quickly now ... I'm in another room now ... I think it is the head teacher's room, Mr F. Mrs P. is there too, shouting and screaming at me, pointing to me ... Mr F. is taking his clothing off ... he stands over me, his long thin penis swinging from side to side, getting bigger and bigger ... Mrs P. is sitting on the floor in front of me, legs spread wide apart ... a big snake is coming out of her pussy ... it's not a snake, it's the arm of an octopus, reaching out for me ... its suction pad is covering my mouth and suddenly I'm being sucked inside the octopus, falling, falling ...

"

This was obviously the repeat of a nightmare she'd had earlier in life, including self-involvement. Although not too common, it is by no means rare for children to have such dreams. In some cases, the dreamer is watching someone else play out a fantasy, so there is a greater degree of objectivity, which is less likely to result in the dreamer carrying through fears incurred by the dream into his/her own sex life.

In those cases where there is subjective involvement in the dream content, there is a greater likelihood of reality identification/-association taking place. Such was the case with Alison, and this session was followed by two similar sessions also resulting in a recurrence of the same dream sequence. This was enough to satisfy me that she was repeating a recurrent dream rather than producing new dreams.

Now I needed to find a solution and I tried to tie the dream in with a symbolic expression which represented Alison's own concept of sex:

> "I want you to relax deeply, Alison, breathing easily and naturally, closing your eyes and descending deep within yourself, to a place where you feel safe and secure, free from tension and stress. A refuge. And

when you're there, I want you to give me
some sort of indication so I will know.

"Good. Now I want you to find something
you can use to represent your feelings
towards sex. A symbol. It doesn't matter
what it is, whether it has a shape, colour, or
what. And when you've found a symbol for
your sexuality I want you to tell me what it
is.
"Okay. Now I want you to drift down,
really deep now, so deep, Alison, you can
feel yourself gently drifting down and
down, down and down, until there is just
no further to go. And when you're as deep
as it's possible for you to go, just give me
some sign so I will know." [At this point
Alison mumbled the word 'cunt'.]

"That's good. Now I'm wondering what
significance or meaning 'cunt' has for you.
Will you think about that and tell me about
it?" [After a long pause, Alison said: "Cunt
is something that sucks you into it and then
kills you."]

"Okay, Alison, I can understand that. You
can feel that way because that is how your

childhood dream depicted it. But you are not a child any longer, and you know just as I know, that a cunt is only a part of a woman's or a girl's body. You know, deep inside you, that a cunt is part of a birth canal, through which babies are born. You also know, deep inside you, that you yourself came out of your own mother's cunt and that you were not sucked into it. You know that, don't you?" [Alison nods]

"Is it possible for you to change that symbol to something else? Something that will make you happier, more satisfied, more fulfilled? Perhaps changing the colour or shape might help. Think about it and see if you would prefer to change that symbol *because that symbol is old, it is no longer appropriate, and it is preventing your happiness.* You don't need it any more."

Alison did give another meaning to that symbol and, in fact, came out of the trance with tremendous relief. She said she had known, while still in trance, that her problem was behind her. I did not see her again with regard to that problem, although she did write to tell me that as soon as she got home she went to her bedroom and immediately explored her own genitalia and, for the first time in her life, finished with masturbation. I saw her three years later to treat her for smoking and she informed me that she was married, had a daughter, and a very happy sex relationship with her husband.

*   *   *

Psychic/Masochist Syndrome Reversal

Some people, men as well as women, go through life first creating and then reproducing circumstances in which they are constantly humiliated and rejected. This enables them to wallow in self-pity, seek sympathy from others, and draw attention to themselves, and generally satisfy a part of themselves while greatly dissatisfying another part.

They seem, to others, never to learn from each experience, and go through life wreaking vengeance – or at least righteous indignation – on successive partners.

Treatment should initially be counselling, and in some cases that will be enough. Merely having a neutral outside telling her that sex should not be a negative, hostile, feelingless affair, but should be based on mature feeling, trust and enjoyment, with each partner contributing positively to the other is often all that is needed.

Sometimes, however, it will be necessary to give much deeper therapy, as in the following case.

Case Study 2:

Sarah B, aged 22.

> "Now there is a part of you that want to prevent you from enjoying sex. And there is another part of you that really wants you to be able to enjoy sex. It is the conflict between these two parts that is causing you problems at the moment. In order to overcome this problem, you are going to have to bring harmony instead of conflict to these different parts.

> "And the way you are going to do this is simply this: I want you to get in touch with that part of you responsible for preventing you from enjoying sex. And when you are in touch, just indicate that to me so that I will know.

> "Okay, Sarah. Now I want you to thank that part for all the good things it has done for

you in the past. Preventing you from enjoying sex has obviously served a useful purpose. It isn't necessary for us to know what that purpose was, but it would be very helpful if we could determine if that purpose is still being served usefully. Or has it now become obsolete, having completed it work?"

In the event that the part agrees that no useful purpose is now being served, it can be asked whether it is now prepared to allow the client to enjoy sex in the future. If the answer is positive, then that is the end of the problem, and the unconscious mind can be told that "from this moment on, you are going to be able to start enjoying sex." If, on the other hand, the part of the mind responsible for sex enjoyment insists that a useful purpose is still being served, then continue along the following lines:

"We are glad to know that a useful purpose is still being served because that shows that you are still being protected. But, is it possible, Sarah, for that same purpose to be served in another way? Could it be served in some way that enables you to still be protected and yet allows you to be able to enjoy sex at the same time. [Wait for an indication.] The part may channel its needs into some other function – like wiggling the little finger, for example – or perhaps it could be satisfied by *creating a new part* whose sole object is to satisfy the part preventing sex from being enjoyable."

Making Things Worse To Make Them Better

Sometimes it is useful to block an intended response in order to release it. Many people quite naturally tend to want what is denied them. The more they are frustrated in satisfying their want, the greater the need becomes. So what starts of as a minor want can, if sufficiently frustrated, quickly become a major want.

This technique is particularly successful when used with *Fantasy Imagery*, in which client is led into a fantasy in which she enters an ideal erotic situation with someone she feels really attracted to. Every time she seems ready to submit sexually, the therapist must force a resistance. By continually restraining her from responding, her determination to respond normally is built up, and finally consented to.

Case Study 3:

Roberta V., aged 28, who had been married but the marriage was annulled because of non-consummation. She told me she'd really wanted to have sex with her husband but just found it impossible to let him touch her. To use her words, "I froze!" Here's how I handled it:

> "Well, Roberta, there is only one way that I know that could get you out of the tangle you're in. The trouble is, it wouldn't suit you. I've used it many times before, with great success, , but it is only suitable for people who would do what I asked them to do. And in your case, I have to tell you that I don't believe you could. So although the method is virtually guaranteed to work, it's not for you."

Obviously, when a carrot like that is held in front of your nose, you'd be pretty annoyed if it wasn't being offered to you. And so it was with Roberta. She couldn't understand why I was so sure she wouldn't be able to do it. I told her because it involved making a promise to my instructions to a 't', and I knew she couldn't do it. The more I told her this. The more she insisted she could.

That, of course, was part of my plan. By holding it out of her reach, she insisted more and more adamantly that she *would* do whatever I demanded Eventually, when I was sure she meant it, I said I would to do if she gave me a solemn promise that she would carry out every single thing I told her to do. She promised. Then I continued:

"Okay, Roberta, now I know this isn't going to be easy for you, but believe me, it's the only way. What you are going to do is this: Tonight, at exactly nine o'clock, you are leaving your flat to go to a pub. You are wearing a very thin blouse, see-through, if you have one, and you are not wearing a bra beneath it. If you don't have one, you'll need to go out and buy one. You're wearing a very tight-fitting, very short skirt. And you're not wearing any underwear beneath it. Nothing.

"You're arriving at this pub, you're going inside, and you are taking stock of everyone inside the pub. You're looking for the most *unattractive* man who is sitting alone. You are going across to him and you're sitting down next to him. Then you are leaning close to him and saying the following words: 'I'm a virgin and I will pay you fifty pounds to take me to a hotel and fuck me!' If he refuses you are demanding to see the manager of the pub, and you are saying to the manager exactly the following words: 'I have offered this man' – pointing to the man – 'fifty pounds to take me to a hotel and fuck me. I don't think you should allow that kind of person into your pub. Either you ask him to leave or I shall have to leave myself.'

"When you have followed these instructions, Roberta, you will be completely cured of your problem. Now don't forget you have promised me you will do it and I shall expect to hear from you tomorrow to that effect."

Of course, I did hear from Roberta the following morning, exactly as I had anticipated. And it had gone approximately along the lines I thought it would. Roberta had gone home in a state of shell-shock, sat down, and cried her eyes out. Then she had picked up the telephone and called her former husband and begged him to come round to see her, promising to let him have sex with her.

You see, I had given Roberta something to do that I knew she couldn't possibly do. And her only way out, after having given me a solemn promise, was to end her problem. And that's what she did. Her former husband went round to see her, they had made love, and Roberta said that they were going to start seeing each other again, and she hoped they would make everything up. Which I later heard they did.

Of course, Roberta would never have taken that route if I hadn't made her promise me. And the only way to extract that promise was by leading her into my carefully laid trap: telling her there was a way, but she wouldn't be able to do it. If I told her without extracting that solemn promise, she would probably have thought me crazy and walked out of my office, and I might never have heard form her again. And, more than likely, she would still have the problem.

Double Indemnity

This is a variation of a technique I use frequently for *Ejaculatory Disorders*. With females suffering from frigidity, it can be used in at least two different ways: by females who are unable to attain sexual pleasure due to hostility towards partner, or due to lack of attraction towards partner.

Sometimes females fake an orgasm to bring a quick end to their ordeal. Therapist:

> "I can fully understand your reasons for that. But what is happening is that you are denying yourself pleasure at the same time. And you don't have to do that! There is a way in which you can pull a fast one over your partner, if that is what you want, and at the same time experience pleasure for yourself without him knowing about it – and thus removing your anxiety about the ordeal.
>
> "When you are going through the motions of faking your orgasm, you can have a *real* orgasm, so he won't know anything about your secret one."

What the client won't realise is that you are pulling a fast one over her in the sense that you are merely changing the context of her orgasm. The fake orgasm is all in her mind *and so is the real one!*

If the client is willing to try that, do an Induction, and let client drift into a normal sex scene with her partner, and go through the usual procedure, faking and *actualising* orgasms simultaneously.

The other technique involves the secret, silent orgasm.

> "I understand that when you don't feel any physical attraction towards a partner it is extremely difficult to show any enthusiasm. But why should you allow him to continue just *using* you without you getting something out of it, too?

> "Well, there is a way in which you can use *him* without hi knowing anything about it. It's called the *silent orgasm*. Instead of you subjecting yourself to this selfishness of his, if you set your mind right before you start, so you can be telling yourself all the time that although he thinks he's using *you*, in fact you are the one who is using *him*. And when you're ready, you can lie there as motionless as you like, but you can be having a wonderful, silent orgasm, made all the sweeter in the knowledge that you are really getting something out of it that he doesn't even know about.

TREATMENTS

Neurotransmitters and amino acids play an important role in sexual arousal.

Norepinephrine, a chemical manufactured in the adrenal medulla is both a hormone and a neurotrans-mitter. Look at its functions, as a neurotransmitter:

- excitatory
- feelings of happiness
- alertness
- motivation
- anti-depressant
- energy
- sexual arousal

Normally, the adrenals would not have a problem making this neurotransmitter, unless there was a deficiency of _L-phenylalanine_, and we have a simple kinesiological test for this, by going to GB 1 on left side only. Weak muscle means we are not providing this synthesiser. Tap point 25 times.

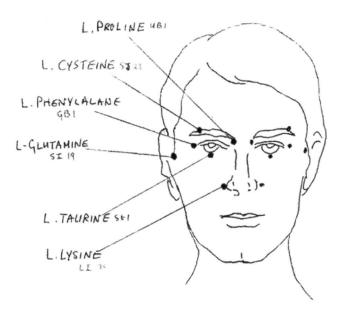

Acetylcholine:

- alertness
- improved memory
- sexual performance
- release of growth hormone

This neurotransmitter is synthesised from choline and acetylCoA, which in turn are catalysed only in the presence of _methionine,_ another amino acid. This can be tested by Tling Liv 1 (lateral aspect of toe 1).

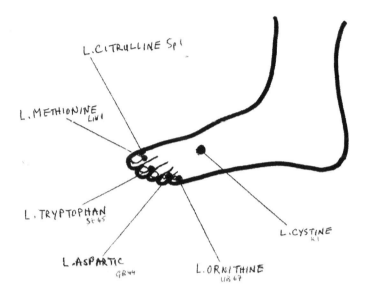

Endorphins, which are opioids, have the following roles:

- mood elevating
- enhancing
- euphoric
- feelings of happiness
- aroused sensitivity
- ability to love
- feelings of pleasure

These endorphins need *dL-phenylalanine*. Remember that for norepinephrine we needed to test for *L-phenylalanine*. Of all the amino acids, phenylalanine is the only one in which the body can use the dL form, which is a mirror-image of the stream of amino acids that make up this protein. All other amino acids can only be used in the L form in the human.

To test for dL-phenylalanine we go to GB 1 again, and test on *both* sides. If weak muscle, then tap on both sides 25 times and retest.

Serotonin, made in the pineal gland functions as hormone and neurotransmitter. It is only in the latter form that we are interested in for this problem.

- Gives emotional stability
- enhances self confidence
-

For this we need a supply of Tryptophan, which we can test for at St 45 (toe 2, lateral aspect), left side only.

Another neurotransmitter, *gamma-amino-butyric acid (GABA)* has a lot of important properties:

- anti stress

- anti anxiety
- anti panic
- anti pain
- promotes feeling of calm
- helps maintain control

GABA needs *L-glutamine*, an amino acid we can test for at SI 19 (anterior to mid-ear), on left side only.

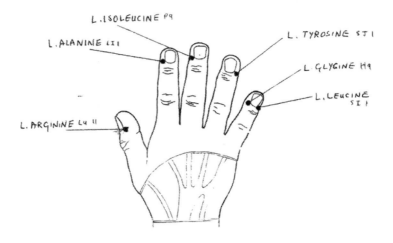

One final hormone, *oxytocin,* which is made in the pituitary gland, enhances:

- sexual arousal
- feelings of emotional attachment
- desire to cuddle

Oxytocin is stimulated by *dopamine*, which requires *L-tyrosine*, which can be tested for at SJ 1 (digit 4, lateral aspect), left side only.

*   *   *

Herbal Treatment

The following list of herbs should be be made up into an infusion (equal parts of each, mixed thoroughly, then 2 teaspoons placed in a cup of boiling water, left to stand for 10-15 minutes, strained, and the liquid sipped):

> Siberian Ginseng root
> Saw Palmetto berries
> Gotu Kola herb
> Echinacea root
> Sarsparilla root
> Garlic bulb
> Chickweed herb

Now we come to the best bit. There has always been a big question, Do we have a sex centre in the brain? The answer is **Yes, we do!**

It took a lot of tracking down, like the lymphatic pump, which I discovered in 1992.

Except that I found the sex centre much earlier, in 1982. It's quite complicated, so I'll keep it as simple as possible.

It is found in area 4 (there are 6 areas of the Sensorimotor Cortex, known as Brodmann's areas, part of the precentral sulcus of the cerebral cortex). Area 4 contains the *giant Betz cells*, named after Vladamir Betz, a Russian scientist (1834-94), which carry sexual messages from the somatic sensory cortex to the thalamus, where they are converted into **action** or **inaction** by the Betz cells.

These can be located by kinesiologically Tling the left and right **posterior eminences**. The left PE tests for *remembered* experiences, the right PE tests for *constructed* desires.

So how can we use this information?

1. Test left PE to see if there are any existing barriers that prevent normal sexual expression. If so, correct by tapping 75-100 times. Retest.
2. Test right PE to see if you have *erected artificial barriers*. Reasons for this are usually due to problems in left PE. This can be tested by 2-pointing left and right PEs together. If a 2-point changes the muscle indicator the problem can be corrected by tapping right PE while Tling the left PE, then tapping left PE while Tling right PE.

Vagus Nerve and VIP

Some interesting research carried out in the US was done by Dr Beverly Whipple on women who had spinal cord injury and who did not thus experience orgasm. The best they could get was a *'phantom orgasm'*.

Using PET scans coupled with MRI scans to provide neuroanatomical localisation, and injecting a tracer – horseradish peroxidase – into the wall of the cervix and uterus, she was able to determine the neurological pathways from the Grafenberg or 'G' spot (a sexually sensitive area felt through the vaginal wall) and the clitoris.

What she found was that though the normal spinal cord pathways were blocked because of the injury or damage, the tracer was found in cell bodies of the nodose ganglion, which is the sensory ganglion of the vagus nerve, confirming that sensory information was carried via the vagus nerve.

Another thing she discovered is that vaginal stimulation caused the release of *vasoactive intestinal peptide*, a neurotransmitter that acts as a vasodilator that carries messages to the brain via the blood-stream. Similarly, clitoral stimulation causes the release of nitric oxide, which travels in the blood and passes messages to the thalamus.

What's particularly interesting about this, kinesiologically speaking, is that VIP is a neurotransmitter form of the hormone *vasopressin,* also known as *anti-diuretic hormone (ADH)* – manufactured in the posterior pituitary gland.

Nitric oxide is formed from arginine as it is broken down by the enzyme *arginase.* And we know we can test for this by Tling L 11 (digit 1, medial aspect) on the left side only. If we get a weak muscle which goes strong when we 2-point with the pineal, or a strong muscle that goes weak with the same 2-point, we can say that this is due to a deficiency in the enzyme arginase. We can correct this by tapping L 11 about 25 times. Then retest.

Before trying the correction above we should test for deficiency of *lysine,* which is similar to arginine but without the probability of bringing on a herpes simplex attack. We can test for this at LI 20 (side of nose) left side only.

Vibrators

It has been known for some time now that the use of vibrators causes *levator ani syndrome* – damage of neuromuscular and neuro-arterial endings of the sensory S1/S5/Coccyx parasympathetic nerves.

Test all the above points and any causing a weak muscle should be stimulated by rotating in a clockwise rotation about 10-15 times.

Female Orgasmic Difficulties

"50% of the women in the U.S. are not having orgasms. If that were true of the male population, it would be declared a national emergency." (Margo St. James)

This is described as a persistent or recurrent delay or absence of an orgasm following the normal sexual excitement phase. It's a surprisingly common female problem, often kept from a partner by the female's ability to 'fake' an orgasm.

The main hormone for libido in both males and females is *testosterone,* the male sex hormone, but also produced in the female adrenal glands.

The amino acid *tyrosine* is a precursor for *dopamine,* which stimulates the libido. We can use kinesiology to check for levels of dopamine, as follows:

Phenylalalanine is another amino acid which is converted into a neuro-transmitter of the same name. This is a relaxant, but also helps deal with stress and agitation. So if the problem can be helped by relieving stress this might help, and can be tested for and stimulated kinesiologically.

Orgasm and the Mind

Female orgasms come about through mental processes. This is confirmed by the fact that females can have orgasmic dreams, hallucinations, during which time there might be no touching of the genitals.

Generally speaking, orgasms do not just happen. Achieving them is a learning process, and if females are unable to achieve them it is usually because they have not learned a suitable technique for doing so.

It also requires concentration, of course. If a female is thinking about what to cook for dinner, or whether she has to do the washing afterwards, it could be difficult to achieve orgasm. Worse, if she is thinking that perhaps her partner is being, or has been, unfaithful towards her, or if she fears his anger or even violence.

I always try to get patients to condition their mind for every important occasion. It can become a habit, and when it does things work much more efficiently.

Sometimes it is necessary to give direct information about the physiological functions of the female genitals, as some females are so mentally dissociated from their body that they don't even know that they can derive   much pleasure through manipulation of the clitoris. Because a female client can be too embarrassed discussing masturbation for herself, a useful technique is to talk about it indirectly:

"This is surprisingly common among young men. Perhaps they've been brought up to believe that even touching the genitals is a sin. As a result, they don't know how to achieve an orgasm through masturbation . And yet they do have orgasms through dreams.

"And sometime they are aware of their penis becoming semi-erect, and then fully erect, and they aren't aware of what it can mean, or what they might do.
And then I tell them that it is all right for them to stimulate themselves manually to orgasm. And it comes as a tremendous relief for them to discover that masturbation is as natural as breathing and eating.

"And we are all half male and half female, anyway. And anything that a male can achieve so a female can achieve. As males can commonly have orgasms through dreams, so can females.

"And as tumescence occurs in the male penis when he becomes sexually aroused, so it also occurs in the female clitoris when she becomes aroused.
And as a man can stimulate his penis until he achieves orgasm, so can a female.

"The wonderful thing about masturbation is that it is Nature's way of allowing us to learn how to prepare ourselves for the sex act with others. When they have learnt how to achieve orgasm, some people, males and females, gradually cease to masturbate. Others prefer to retain this practice. It doesn't really matter."

Change of Motivation

Some prostitutes and some nymphomaniacs find it difficult or even impossible to achieve an orgasm. The reasons here are quite different from other cases, the first using sex merely as a means of exploitation, the latter in a fruitless search for a satisfaction which is never achieved.

To change either of these types requires a change of motivation. Clearly there is a conflict of requirements otherwise they would not be coming for treatment. On the one hand they want to achieve an orgasm; on the other, they want to exploit men, either for money for an unrealistic ideal. And what they are doing is completely incongruous: they are having plenty of sex and they are not enjoying it one little bit.

It is not a question of techniques because both types probably know more about various techniques than do any of us. It is a question of mind set: they are indulging in sex, not for pleasure, but for another reason which has nothing to do with pleasure.

It is important here to work at a level beneath awareness because they have already demonstrated that awareness exacerbates the problem rather than ameliorating it. Working beneath awareness can be done metaphorically:

> "Go back in time, way back to the time when you were a very small child. So small that you could only crawl along the floor. You could see other, bigger people walking

in the room but you could still only crawl. And you made up your mind that you were going to walk, too.

"But first you had to be able to stand. So you tried to stand, by first pulling yourself up the leg of a chair, falling down several times in the early stages until finally you could do it, not only when holding on to something but even without using your hands at all.

"And then you took your first step. And came crashing down with a bump. But it didn't deter you, and you pulled yourself up again, stood up, and took another step, tentatively. You fell down again.

"But as you repeated this over and over again you managed to go from one step to two, and from two steps to three, until you were walking all around the room without falling once.

"You became so good at it that before long you were able to walk and run without even having to look down at your feet to make sure you were going in the right direction. You could climb stairs and you could go down stairs without any difficult at all.

"And a few years later you went to school. You'd noticed that grown-ups, and even a lot of other children, could pick up a book and all the little things that were written on a page seemed to make sense to them. They called it reading. And you wanted to learn to read. But first you had to learn what all the little letters meant.

"At first it made no sense at all to you. How could you tell the difference between a p and a q? You thought you'd never learn it, but you were determined, because the rewards were worthwhile.

"So you struggled on until eventually it all clicked into place. And the same with reading. You wanted to learn to read, to turn all those words into sounds, and although it was a struggle you made it.

"Now, today, you have no difficult in walking, or reading. You don't have to watch foot as you come down the stairs. In fact, if you tried you're more likely to stumble over your feet. And when you're reading, you don't have to study each letter that makes up a word. You just read in chunks of letters and perhaps even in chunks of words.

"You did all these things, despite the difficulties, because you wanted to. You wanted to be able to do things that other people seem to take for granted. Things that added to the quality of life and to the pleasures of life.

"Yet in a strange and curious way, you never quite managed to master the pleasures of sex. You know, when we read a book written in our own language, we read across the page from left to right. Yet the Chinese read from right to left. Think what would have happened if we tried to read our books as the Chinese read theirs. It wouldn't make any sense to us.

"But there are people, in this country, who actually try to read a book from right to left, because that is the way they decided to learn. As a result, they can't make any sense out of a page and they can't get any real pleasure from reading a book.

"These people are actually quite intelligent, and there is a part of them that actually knows they are depriving themselves of pleasure, yet they might not know why.

"Perhaps they are afraid of something. Yet they have no need to be afraid of something which comes naturally for most people.... "

There is a combination of learning behaviour, motivation, and metaphorical change in that example. I always make a point of not trying to explain meanings to a client when doing metaphorical work. It is important that their own mind should evaluate and extract any meaningful phrases and apply it.

Questionnaire

Outline of Dysfunction

1. Have you at any time achieved an orgasm?
2. At what point were you unable to achieve orgasm through intercourse?
3. Can you attain orgasm now through masturbation?
4. Do you sometimes indicate to partner that you have had an orgasm even when you have not?
5. Are you able to achieve an orgasm in some situations and not in others?
6. What seems to prevent you from having an orgasm?

7. Does your partner show concern when you do not have an orgasm?
8. Are you afraid to 'let yourself go'?
9. Are you able to discuss any problems or difficulties with partner?
10. Do you and your partner indulge in sexual foreplay?

Upbringing and Childhood

1. Were you brought up with strong religious convictions?
2. Do you have strong religious convictions now?
3. Do you have any convictions that *sex* is either bad or dirty, and should only be indulged in for procreative purposes?
4. Were you brought up strictly by parents?
5. Did your mother ever talk to you about sex?
6. Where and when did you first learn about masturbation?
7. Were you ever warned against masturbation? By whom?
8. Were you ever caught indulging in any sexual activity as a child?

Sexual Learning

1. How did you first learn about sexual intercourse?
2. What was your initial reaction?
3. In masturbation do you use your fingers or some object?
4. Have you tried using a vibrator? Does this help?
5. Do you like your partner to touch your genitals?
6. Are you able to communicate openly with partner about your sexual likes and dislikes?
7. Is your partner sometimes/often/never able to bring you to orgasm through (a) coitus (b) manual manipulation (c) oral stimulation
8. Describe a typical sex encounter with partner:

Pregnancy

1. Do you or your partner take contraceptive precautions?
2. Have you had an abortion or miscarriage?
3. Do you worry about becoming pregnant?
4. Does your partner worry about you becoming pregnant?
5. Has your sexual attitude changed as a result of pregnancy?

Relationships

1. Are you still sexually attracted towards partner?
2. Were you ever sexually attracted towards partner?
3. At what point did your attraction change?
4. Do you trust your partner?
5. Are you satisfied that your partner stimulates you adequately?
6. Are you afraid of your partner in any way?
7. Has your partner tried to help you to orgasm other than intercourse? Describe:

Self-Punishment and Sexual Reversal

Test muscle and say,

"Do I want pleasure?"

"Do I want punishment?"

Obviously, a sexually-healthy person would test strong for the former and weak for the latter. But the female who is *sexually reversed* is different.

Say,

"To deny yourself an orgasm is a form of self-punishment. Obviously, there was a good reason why you felt you deserved punishing – perhaps at an unaware level. It is not important that you or I should know what that reason is. But there comes a time when punishment should cease, when the price has been paid in full. And I want to ask you now, Has your price been paid in full?"

Test muscle. If strong, ask, "Can I stop punishing myself now, and start to have orgasms?" Test muscle. If strong, that is end of treatment.

If answer to the first question is weak, then follow up with a supplementary question:

"When will my price be paid in full? One week's time? Two week's time?" and so on. Test muscle with each question until getting getting a strong response.

Or you could say, "Could the punishment be reduced so that I have an orgasm on some occasions and not on others?" Test muscle.

Side Effects of Dep Provera

Depo Provea is the name of a birth control injection – instead of taking a contraceptive pill every day, you get an injection 3 times a year.

Women are always told that it's perfectly safe, but look at these side effects, already experienced by a growing number of women:

1. up to 25 kilos weight gain
2. extreme excitability, nervousness
3. panic attacks, paranoia
4. shortness of breath
5. great loss of libido
6. painful intercourse
7. severe lack of lubrication
8. lowered immune system
9. loss of hair
10. unwanted hair on breasts, toes, face
11. violent headaches
12. extremely sore, stiff muscles all over body
13. blurry vision
14. dizziness
15. inability to bend over
16. severe neck and shoulder pain
17. breast tenderness and pains
18. heart palpitations
19. chronic sinus and yeast infections
20. concentration and memory problems
21. acne
22. suicidal thoughts because daily debilitating pain too much to bear

Now let's take a look at what happens when you start having these shots. Progestin (a pseudo-progesterone) poisons the liver, disables the ovarian functions, negatively disturbs the brain's dopamine, acetylcholine nervous systems and slows down thyroid functions, resulting in moodswings, depression, weight gain, vaginal dryness, intercourse or penetration pain, loss of libido, breast tenderness, tiredness, fatigue, joint pains, muscular cramps, blurry vision, dizziness, yeast infection, immune weakness, headaches, menstrual interruption and so on. All the symptoms reported above.

Generally, birth control shots or implants produce more and broader damage than the pills do (and they're bad enough!). The common problems of the birth control drugs are the increasing production of prolactin (a hormone made in the pituitary gland, which inhibits orgasms) and the decreasing production of dopamine and testosterone due to the poisoned liver.

The liver has to deactivate all the other functions and to work extremely hard to detoxify this toxin.

Here's how progestin works:

It binds into the progesterone receptors to trigger the brain's Progesterone Negative Feedback

Controller in the hypothalmus-pituitary-ovarian axis, and refuses to go away once it takes over the receptors. Its behaviours are like street drugs, but fortunately it's not addictive.

The brain's/nervous systems are then poisoned, and have to shut down the entire ovarian functions which are supposed to produce oestrogen, progesterone and androstenedione/-testosterone/DHEA to regulate the menstrual cycle and sexual/orgasmic functions.

Now her body is flooded by the synthetic (or fake) progesterone. The effects can last for several years from just one shot.

The most effective treatment is to detoxify the liver and brain's nervous systems.

The Use of Vibrators

Do they have sex shops near you? I don't know if one can buy vibrators from anywhere else, but I presume everyone knows what a vibrator is and how and why it's used.

What most people don't know is whether or not it can actually cause damage. And the answer is yes. Here's what it can do:

- it abrades the clitoral and G-spot nerves and tissue
- can also damage the urethral and bladder's parasympathetic nerves that control urinary incontinence, resulting in urethral female ejaculation.

The best treatment I can suggest is the homeopathic HH 960 Clitostore, which is specifically designed to repair damage to the clitoris and soft vaginal tissue (including the G-spot).

The Oriental Approach

The Chinese (and the Indians) have had a very enlightened approach to sex for thousands of years, whereas the Occidentals are only in the last 40-50 years approaching enlightenment.

One of the features of their approach is that the female is equally entitled to enjoy sex . Hundreds of techniques were developed to help women achieve their orgasm. One of their discoveries was the G-spot and the orgasmic epicentre. They claim that in order for a female to orgasm there must be a degree of G-spot engorgement.

This engorgement can be verified by checking with a finger. The underside of the finger is inserted into the vagina just below the clitoris. The G-spot zone is extruded like an upside-down ridge hanging over the vaginal ceiling.

The epicentre is much deeper inside – too far for a finger to reach, and is placed just above and slightly behind the cervix.

They believe that the Orgasmic Wave Energy is pumped out by the contraction of the uterus. The pelvic cavity burns up testosterone which then traps and resonates the orgasmic waves.

The main acupuncture channel for this is the Ren (Conception Vessel). Ren 2 directly influences the clitoris, which can be stimulated by lightly massaging Ren 2 in a clockwise direction about 25 times.

Ren 3 and Ren 4 both stimulate the burning of testosterone in the pelvic cavity, also in a clockwise direction.

SELF DESTRUCT

Let's talk about this concept in which a person seems to obey some hidden, internal command that works against that person's best interests. We have available a terrific technique for correcting this problem.

Why would a person want to sabotage their own best interests? It doesn't make sense, you might think. Yet the truth is that people, for different reasons, do exactly that. Fortunately, we have a brand new treatment which is one of the most powerful treatments in kinesiology.

Nothing happens by accident. There is a compelling reason behind every act, every behaviour we have. Not surprisingly, we have to go to the brain both to understand and also to treat.

First, I believe that all self-destruct commands come about because of something that was said to us at an earlier time in our lives. Think back, for a moment, and try and recall if any of these commands have been given to you in the past:

"Shut up"

"You're just a child"

"You're nothing"

"You're stupid"

"Grow up"

"You'll never amount to anything"

"You're a bad person"

"You're not a nice person"

"You can never remember anything"

"You're dumb"

"You don't know anything"

"You're worthless"

"You're useless"

and so on.

There are two things about these commands:

1. they all start with the word 'you' or 'you're' (you are)

2. because they are words, they are received by that part of the brain that deals with speech sensory input, which is called *Wernicke's area*. Would you believe it, this is the point that we use for testing the hypothalamus.

This now opens up a whole new understanding of why so many of the treatments we've used in the past work so well. We knew they worked, now we know why they work.

Now let's think about the significance of this. The negative commands are being picked up by the brain's speech sensory centre, Wernicke's area, and all the commands – from another person, who may be parent, sibling, peer, teacher, etc. - start with **you**.

In the past, haven't we always thought in terms of **I**?

"I am nothing"

"I am stupid"

"I should grow up"

"I am being childish"

"I'm a bad person"

"I'll never amount to anything"

"I'm not a nice person"

"I can never remember anything"

"I'm dumb"

"I don't know anything"

"I'm worthless"

"I'm useless"

"I can never please anybody"

These repetitive negative commands, received in the Wernicke's area, are recorded in the limbic brain, and because they are *hurtful* at the time, are imbued with emotions which make them stick.

One-off negative commands might hurt a little at the time but are usually forgotten or shrugged off. It is the repetition of these negative commands – particularly if they are picked up by others and repeated (which forms a reinforcement) – which then create lesions in the speech *motor* centre – *Broca's area*.

It is this area which activates or inhibits action. And this position is at a level of the hypothalmic point but in front of the ear instead of behind it. If you feel around, and do it gently because the area is quite tender or sensitive, you'll find a slight niche.

So now we know a little bit more than we knew before, so we are ready to start doing some testing. And the key to testing is finding the *exact wording* of the original negative command that created the lesion in the first place.

1) Begin by asking person if they have any knowledge of a command. They might know, or it might have become buried beneath all other kinds of debris piled on top. But if they know it's a help, because you can test them on it. If they don't know, ask them which area of their life is giving them problems, then try going through a variety of negative commands, trying to seek the appropriate one. Remember, you have to find the **exact** words that caused the lesion.

2) To test, ask person to say the words – aloud or silently, depending on their choice – while they turn their eyes upwards and obliquely to the left. Remember, they have to start each negative command with "You or You're" and not with "I", because that is how they received it in the first place. In addition, they must TL the Wernicke's area point, first on the left side only. If you get a weak muscle you can proceed.

3) We now go to the *significance centre* on the left side, and TL with eyes still looking up and obliquely to the left. Test. If muscle goes weak, this is confirmation that we have now found the negative command or phrase that the brain is converting to self-destruct. If we do not get a weak muscle on **both** of these tests we can conclude that we have not yet got the correct negative command and must start again.

4) Now to test for treatment we go to the right side of the brain, to the **Significance Centres**, and retest exactly as before except with the eyes looking up and obliquely to the right. The muscle should now be strong.

Treatment is in three phases:

1. inhale deeply with eye (closed) looking up to right obliquely. Place a finger gently on eye lid, pushing very lightly in same direction. Lift finger during exhalation.
2. Inhale deeply with eye (closed) looking horizontally to right side. Again, during inhalation phase, place finger lightly on eyelid pushing in same direction.
3. Inhale deeply with eye (closed) looking obliquely down to right sidde. Place finger on eyelid as before, this time pushing gently obliquely down to right.

Retest as before, Tling Wernicke's area while repeating the negative command. Muscle will be strong if the negative command has itself been negated.

It may be necessary to search for another negative command. If found, repeat above test and treatment regime.

More About Vibrators

The use of vibrators, biking and horse-riding, can all damage the superficial nerves of the clitoris and labia. This can affect arousal normally leading to an orgasm, and cause a fall-back on G-spot and Epicentre orgasm – which is a different kind of orgasm. (Can use **Clitoroil** treatment)

Orgasm physically depends on the ratio between testosterone and oestrogen. With friction (through masturbation or intercourse), testosterone becomes electrically charged and heats the clitoral and pudendal nerves when it is burned and converted to *dihydrotestosterone* (DHT). Oestrogen cools the nerves (like a water-cooling system), which causes them to discharge – creating the Orgasmic Wave. Too much oestrogen has the effect of over-cooling the process (going off the boil, so to speak), and can also lead to thickening of the tissue thickness surrounding the G-spot, thus reducing sexual stimulation to that point.

Women with high oestrogen levels should be stimulated at the Epicentre, which is equivalent to the male prostate. Stimulating the Epicentre with a rhythmic pressure of about 1 KSC (kilos per square centimetre) can trigger an orgasm even when oestrogen levels are very high. That is why labour can give women an orgasm providing there is no significant pain.

Qi-Gong Breathing

This is a method which can help power the brain's acetylcholine, dopamine and serotonin nervous functions with the essential hormones and nutrients. The acetylcholine and PNS functions are responsible for the promotion of penile/G-spot/clitoral erection and sizes (due to release of 2nd n't Nitric Oxide and the arterial dilator cGMP (cyclic Guanosine monophosphate) and mutually associated with the local secretion of the relaxant hormone prostaglandins E-1 (PG-E1) in the local tissues and arterial walls for arterial dilation during lovemaking, in conjunction with the biological action of testosterone and DHEA in the hormone receptors in the brain and sex organs.

The autorhythmic fibres of the Epicentre (the orgasmic pacemaker) are ignited when the dopamine/SNS circuits are bioelectrically triggered by the over-erection (over-stress) of the urethral spongy tissues and nerves in synchronizing with the sudden surge of oxytocin released from the pituitary.

If you have a proper erection of the urethral/vaginal spongy tissues, an intensified stimulation will signal the pituitary to release a burst of orgasmic hormone oxytocin, the brain will switch the autonomic nervous function from parasympathetic erection to sympathetic orgasm, and at the same time, the dopamine-norepinephrine-epinephrine (stress hormone) will burst.

Thus, the ultimate uterine/vaginal contraction will be initiated by the orgasmic pacemaker and the orgasmic wave energy will be radiated out of the pelvic cavity, running up to the heart, lungs, forehead, and then the brain's cerebral cortex (your conscious controller) via the frontal energy path (Ren or Conception Vessel of the acupuncture network) so that you will lose conscious control of your body and your heavy breathing, crying, moaning, and movement of body parts ar synchronising with the 0.8 seconds beating rate of the uterine/vaginal contraction.

This whole process can be totally enhanced by what I call the Qi-Gong Breathing Cycle. Exerting an inhaling (qi) pressure against the bladder is to turn the bladder's sensory-parasympathetic nervous circuits for over-riding the prostate/uterine sensory-sympathetic (ejaculation and orgasmic) circuits. So does contracting the coccyx.

The bioelectric recharge is done by burning testosterone in the local tissues. The pelvic cavity is the normal hormone reception centre. The tissues contain a lot of testosterone and oestrogen receptors that can trap a lot of testosterone and oestrogen respectively. The Epicentre (the area between prostate and bladder in men and between cervix and bladder in women) is the testosterone reception centre. Burning testosterone there promotes libido and drives orgasm high during sexual activity.

During this Qi Gong Breathing Exercise, the bladders PNS nerves discharge bioelectric flow into the Ren circuit, and when you are contracting the coccygeal muscle the bioelectric flow moves across the anus from CV-1 (between the anus and scrotum or between anus and vagina) to Du-1, where the bioelectric energy partially flows into the Du channel and partially feeds the sensory nerves around the coccyx.

Then the bioelectric current in the sensory nerves is split into two parts in the inter-neuron switches-splitters inside the S-1 to S-5 and Coccyx. A large part of energy is coupled in the spinal cord nerves/CNS to the brain's cerebral cortex (sensory and then motor areas for response; the rest of the energy is reflected back to the genital area through the S-1 to S-5 and CO parasympathetic motor nerves that drive the erection and engorge-ment blood pressures from the pubis-penis (clitoris and vaginal/urethral spongy tissues) groins to the coccyx. This means you activate the orgasmic/ejaculation circuits.

The Exercise

Think about having an orgasm-ejaculation.

Test muscle. May be weak.

Contract coccygeal muscle during the in-breath and relax during out-breath.

Do 3 cycles, then test muscle.

DYSPAREUNIA

Dyspareunia means painful or difficult intercourse, as distinct from vaginismus, in which painful muscular spasms usually prevent intercourse from taking place. Unlike vaginisimus, which is mostly psychogenic in origin, dyspareunia is frequently due to some physical abnormality.

Organic or physical causes may include:

Vagina:
- an intact hymen, or irritated or bruised remnants of hymenal ring
- unprotected scar area at junction of vaginal mucosa and perineal body, often due to childbirth, sometimes to rape or forced sex
- Bartholin gland area may be enlarged at gland base
- after menopause labia and vagina may have lost some elasticity and become shrunken, leading to pain on intromission
- vulval infection
- vulvodynia (vulva hypersensitive to touch)

Clitoris:

- smegma beneath clitoral hood can cause chronic irritation and burning
- adhesions anchoring clitoral glans to hood can cause severe pain
- clitoris sometimes over-sensitive as result of heavy-handedness

Vaginal Barrel:

- lack of adequate lubrication leads to friction and chronic irritation (check here for penetration after rectal penetration)
- vaginal infection from that or clothing material
- superficial or deep lacerations due to foreign object inserted into vagina
- chronic fungal infection can cause severe irritation or pain
- ovarian cysts
- prolapsed ovaries or uterus
- vaginal prolapse

Treatment for these should normally be carried out under professional supervision, and may include contraceptive creams, jellies and suppositories, foams or foam tablets. (Care should be taken to see that no sensitivity occurs as reaction to any chemicals used.) There is occasional irritation from use of rubber contraceptives and diaphragms, so monitoring when rubber items used is advisable.

Lack of secretion due to inadequate sexual foreplay is sometimes responsible for dyspareunia, and this can usually be determined through questionnaire.

Not all dyspareunia problems are are due to physical reasons, however. There can be a lack of sexual interest in partner, fear of pregnancy, inadequate techniques. There can also be a secondary gain factor associated with this condition and one needs to be wary of this, since it induces a female to hold on to her symptoms in order to avoid any kind of sexual contact with their partner.

All females with dyspareunia are not sexually cold, and some are quite able to achieve orgasm through clitoral stimulation, cunnilingus, and sometimes even through coitus despite the pain.

Where the symptoms do appear to be psychogenic in origin it is usually advisable to see both partners together. The interpersonal relationship islikely to be at the root, and a full round table discussion concerning the relationship itself, the techniques used, and any other factors which seem relevant, can often lead to successful counselling. It frequently reveals that the husband/partner himself has sexual inadequacies which need treatment, and these should be given separately.

Inadequate lubrication is often a factor, and this may be due to insufficient foreplay. The pain experienced is often only apparent during penetration or attempted penetration, and coital techniques might need to be adjusted here in order to facilitate the initial intromission: a suitable jelly (P-Y is often used because it does not clog and is sterile), and a pillow placed beneath the buttocks changes the angle of the vagina and makes penetration easier.

The penetration itself should be slow, considerate, and combined with a display of tenderness and care towards the female; any attempt at creating any friction at this stage should be avoided.

Treatments

Infections are usually treated with antibiotics, and some excellent homeopathic remedies exist for this purpose. Some herbal remedies also have mild antiobitic effects.

Any local inflammations would be best treated with anti-inflammatories, and again they can homeopathic, if preferred.

Dryness of the vagina is usually caused by dysfunctional Bartholin's glands, which have small opening inside the outer labia. They can be tested kinesiologically by Tling the local site. A weak muscle indicates a problem, and this can be corrected homeopathically, or by lightly stimulating the Bartholin's gland in a clockwise direction.

Lactation sometimes causes this problem as a result of increased prolactin. An intravaginal homeopathic oestrogen cream can be used for that, and also for postmenopausal vaginal atrophy.

System Restore

It follows that painful intercourse could not have existed prior to the first, or later, experience of intercourse. So we need to try and establish that first time, and we can do that, hopefully, by asking client to go back in time to the first coital experience and test muscle.

If muscle is weak, we can assume that that was the first experience. To proceed from there we ask them to go back to that experience while we conduct a series of further tests:

- Was the actual entry painful because it was done in an uncaring way? Test.

- Was the size of penis too large? Test.
- Was force used? Test.
- Were you an unwilling participant? Test.

Depending on the answer, it may then be possible to go back to a point just befre that first experience and say to the client, "You have never experienced painful intercourse and you know that it is not necessary for intercourse to be painful, now or in the future. When you return to the present, you are finding that all future sexual experiences can be without pain.

Questionnaire

1. Where is the pain located?
2. When is the onset of pain (before, entry, vaginal, deep or after)
3. What is the chronologic history? If multiple pain sites, which came first?
4. Is it situational or positional?
5. Has it been lifelong or acquired?
6. Are there any other sexual dysfunctions, such as arousal, lubrication or orgasmic difficulties?
7. What treatments have been attempted?

Potential Gynecologic Causes?

1. Are there vaginal symptoms, including discharge, burning or itching?
2. Is there an obstetric delivery history of lacerations or other trauma?
3. Is there an abdominal or genitourinary surgical or radiation history?
4. Has the patient had prior XXXynaecologic diagnoses, including endometriosis, fibroids or chronic pelvic pain?
5. What is the patient's current contraception method and is there any history of intrauterine device use?

Explore Potential Medical Causes

1. Is there evidence or history of chronic disease?
2. What are the patient's medications: alternative, prescribed, over-the-counter?
3. Is there alcohol or drug use?
4. Does the patient experience bowel or bladder symptoms?
5. Is there evidence of skin disorders, such as eczema, psoriasis, or other dermatitis?

Obtain Psychosocial Information

1. What is the patient's view of the problem?
2. Has the problem been present in other relationships?
3. Are the partners able to discuss the problem? If so, what actions have they tried?
4. Is there any history of ssexual or physical abuse?
5. To what extent are other life stressors a factor?
6. Is there evidence of depression or anxiety disorders?
7. What would be considered a satisfactory treatment outcome?

TREATMENTS

Homoeopathic

There are a number of physical or organic problems which can cause dyspareunia. These include any of the following, which can be tested for in the *Sex Kinesiology* Test Kit, together with remedies.

1. Anal fissure
2. Bartholinitis
3. cystitis
4. gonorrhoea
5. haemorrhoids (external)

6. haemorrhoids (internal)
7. inflammation of the hymen (vaginal membrane)
8. inflammation of the nervus pudendus
9. inflammation of the urethra (urethritis)
10. labial oedema
11. metritis
12. ovarian inflammation (left)
13. ovarian inflammation (right)
14. perineal tear
15. prolapse of ovary (left)
16. prolapse of ovary (right)
17. vulvitis

Vaginal Dryness

Vaginal wetness reflects the oestrogen levels, and has nothing to do with orgasm. Younger women tend to get wet more easily than older women and are thus more likely to experience clitoral orgasm, whereas the older woman is more likely to experience a vaginal orgasm.

The vaginal lining that covers and protects the g-spot and Epicentre, is thinner for the middle-aged woman. The thicker the vaginal lining the more the orgasmic difficulty the women will encounter.

But the most common 'dryness' problem concerns the secretions from the Bartholins glands, which are situated in the labial folds. When these fail to secrete, or secretions are inadequate, the vulva itself becomes very dry and any kind of friction or rubbing can be painful.

Tests

TL the gland (see diagram) and test muscle. Weak indicator shows lack of secretion.

To treat this, rotate in clockwise direction about 25 times then retest.

If over-secretion, rotate in counter-clockwise direction about 10-15 times then retest.

Clues to Diagnosis

Pain Descriptors
1. Location—entry versus deep pain differential
2. Onset—entry versus deep pain (pain after intercourse points to pelvic congestion)
3. Pruritic or burning pain—vaginitis; vulvodynia; atrophy or inadequate lubrication
4. Aching—pelvic congestion
5. single/multiple sites—e.g. Patient had initial viginitis or other pain with entry, then developed vulvodynia or inadequate

lubrication from decreased arousal resulting from pain expectation

6. Situational/generalised—occurs only with certain partners, situations or with all encounters
7. Positional—deep-thrusting pain may be minimised with use of woman-superior positions or other position changes
8. Lifelong/acquired—

Historical

1. Other sexual dysfunctions?—arousal disorders may affect lubrication
2. previous treatments—patient's perspective on the problem
3. Vaginal symptoms;discharge/odour —vaginitis
4. History of STD—adhesions and complications of pelvic inflammatory disease
5. Obstetric history; lacerations, traumas—postpartum dyspareunia (minority have pain at site of repair), adhesions, pelvic relaxation
6. Abdominal/genitourinary surgery, or radiation—post-surgical changes; vaginal stricture or shortening; trauma to structures; inadequate lubrication

7. Endometriosis, fibroids, or chronic pelvic pain—pain may be difficult to separate; often deep pain
8. Contraception—(condoms, intrauterine device, gels, foams, sponge, caps, diaphragm); risk of pelvic inflammatory disease; trauma/irritation

Possible Medical Causes

1. Chronic diseases—diabetes; Behçet's syndrome
2. Medications—decreased arousal and inadequate lubrication
3. Bowel or bladder symptoms—genitourinary disorders; irritable bowel syndrome
4. Skin disorders—vulvar dystrophies, sensitivities to lotions or other topical agents
5. DSM-IV—Diagnostic and Statistical Manual of Mental Disorders, 4th Edition—STD (sexually transmitted disease), HSV= herpes simplex virus; HPV= human papilloma virus

CAUSES of DYSPAREUNIA

Abdominal Disorders

- chronic pelvic inflammatory diseases
- diabetes
- endometriosis

Congenital Factors

- Hymenal stenosis
- vaginal agenesis
- vaginal duplication
- Vaginal septation

Gastrointestinal Disorders

- chronic constipation
- diverticular disease
- haemorrhoids
- inflammatory bowel disease
- proctitis

Lubrication Inadequacy

- abuse (past or present)
- arousal disorders
- insufficient foreplay
- medications
- progesterone-only contraceptives
- vaginal atrophy

Pelvic Scarring

- episiotomy

- surgery

Psychological Factors

- anxiety
- depression

Trauma

- physical
- psychological

Urologic Disorders

- cystitis (acute or chronic)
- interstitial cystitis
- lichen sclerosis
- urethral diverticulum
- urethritis

Uterine and Ovarian Disorders

- adenomyosis
- leiomyoma of the uterus
- ovarian mass
- prolapsed adnexa

Vaginal Disorders

- atrophic vaginitis
- vaginismus
- vaginitis

Vulvar Disorders

- irritation from chemicals
- infection with herpes simplex virus
- hypertrophic vulvar dystrophy
- lichen sclerosis
- vulvitis
- vulvodynia
- vestibulitis

ACUVI

Have patient lie prone on the floor while holding a vial – Dyspareunia— in her hand

Apply acupressure technique. Close hands with thumbs extended. Starting at the base of the neck of the patient, place thumbs on patient, approximately 3 cm on either side of the vertebrae. With deliberate and firm pressure, the thumbs are pressed directly into the back at each vertebra site.

The procedure is then repeated, except that this time the patient is asked to lie in a supine positine, and pressure is only applied to Urinary

Bladder 65 for about 10-15 seconds, while the patient still holds vial.

The patient continues to hold vial for fifteen minutes after treatment is finished.

Vaginismus

Vaginismus is a severe contraction of vaginal muscles prior to penetration, usually causing considerable pain and chronic tension.

Primary vaginismus is organic in origin, while _Secondary vaginismus_ has a psychogenic basis.

It is essential to have a physical examination before treatment can be planned. Physical factors could include:

- Congenital deformation of the vagina
- Introital damage or infection (to entrance of vagina)
- Retroversion of the uterus
- Pelvic tumor
- Polyps

- Cervicitis (inflammation of the cervix uteri . neck of the uterus)
- Tender episiotomy scar (surgical incision in vulva for obstetric purposes)
- Kraurosis vulvae (dry glistening condition of the mucous membrane of the vulva, characterised by intense itching and constitutional disturbance from loss of sleep)
- Urethral caruncle (small bright red growth at entrance of the urethra. It is very painful, and bleeds readily on being touched)

Despite this list of organic causes, most cases of vaginismus are psychogenic, and commonly include any of the following:

- Faulty psychosexual development
- Fear of being too small
- Defence against contraception, often due to religious convictions)
- Hostility against partner
- Phobic reaction to penetration by a foreign object
- Fear of pregnancy
- Reaction to partner having a sexual dysfunction mother's command (as a child) to always keep her legs crossed

There is often a strong secondary gain, with the client wanting to be helped, yet at the same time being frightened because once cured she no longer has a defence against intercourse, which is what she fears. In some cases, it is possible to trace the condition to a single frightening experience, which thus created a phobic condition.

Partners frequently need treatment themselves as there is a tendency for a man to develop secondary impotence as a direct result of his partner's vaginismus. .

Counselling is often a good first step in treatment, especially when there is a need to correct faulty conceptions, i.e. religious misconceptions, Victorian-style upbringing ("Close your eyes and think of Jesus"), or childhood fears of sex.

I have found in practice that a frequent factor causing vaginismus is the result of indecent exposure by an adult man to a small girl, in which what seems to her like an enormous penis. Quite naturally, when the girl learns – if she doesn't already know – that intercourse is penile entry to her vagina, it is not surprising that she finds it a frightening proposition.

Counselling for that kind of belief/fear usually needs to be followed up by something more powerful than just counselling; indeed, a female might not be conscious of the reason. Sometimes, an extremely painful introduction to sex might create a phobic anxiety, in which she believes that all sex will be as painful as that first time.

Vaginismus may be employed as a defence against having to endure intercourse, or it might be a way of demonstrating hostility towards partner. Either case should show up through the questionnaire, and in either case a strategy of treatment can be prepared.

Treatments

Anchoring

This is a technique I developed for *Neurolinguistic Kinesiology (NK)*, but in this case we are going to use it in a different manner. A simple method of dealing with a phobic anxiety is not merely to take it away – the client might well have a psychological need for it – but to offer another choice, or choices.

Let's take an example:

Maria has vaginal spasms because she has a terrible fear of being penetrated by a foreign object, i.e. penis. Now, instead of removing the fear of penises altogether, after inducing a light trance we can say:

> "And you are finding, Maria, that whenever you are in a situation of facing sexual intercourse with a man whose penis is at least 30 cm long [anchor], you are experiencing painful vaginal spasms, and intercourse is becoming impossible. But on all other occasions [anchor], when your partner has a penis of less than 30 cm, there is no need for you to feel any painful spasms at all. In fact, you are finding yourself capable of really enjoying sex [anchor] with a partner whose penis is less than 30 cm long."

Laying the first anchor establishes a time when the vaginal spasms she has already been encountering may return. And since our 30 cm man is so remote, the anxiety is never likely to return. Remember that a phobic anxiety is only a learned response that is aroused whenever confronted with a particular stimuli. Whenever that stimuli is presented the response is always the same. We additionally anchor the other two *overwhelming* anchors that on all other occasions she is going to find intercourse pleasurable.

Changing Memory

One of the great things about people with phobic anxieties is that they're easy to treat. The reason they're easy to treat is that they're easy to influence. The very fact that they have a phobic response to a set stimuli pattern is proof of that. The vast majority of us can't achieve that, which means that we're so easy to influence. So when we get clients who say that they always respond in the same way to the same stimuli, i.e. painful vaginal spasms, we know that it should not be difficult to change that response.

Anchoring is one way, Changing Memory is another, more subtle way, We want to get the client onto her time line:

> "So which direction is the future [wait for her to point] and which direction is the past [wait for her to point]. Okay, Maria, and I want you to go back in time to the very first occasion when you experienced those painful spasms. Go all the way back, and I shall be going back with you. So you'll still hear my voice and be aware of my presence, but you will be there in mind and in body, exactly as it was then. And you

will hear my voice although I won't be there with you. You can see everything the way it was. Nod your head when you are there. [When client nods, test muscle. Should be weak]

"Will you tell me where you are and who you are with? [wait] Can you describe in detail what happened? [wait]

"Okay. Now I want you to go through all that again, except that this time, instead of being there, I want you to stand outside the experience – above your time line – and *watch yourself* undergoing that experience once again.

"And while you're watching it, I want you to realise that there is something about yourself that you know but you don't know that you know. And as soon as you find out what it is you know but don't know that you know, you can the whole experience becomes pleasant and enjoyable. And when it's finished, please nod. [Wait, then test muscle. Should now be strong]

"Now Maria, can you tell me what happened when you were watching yourself?" [wait]

If the experience was a pleasant one, as suggested, then bring client forward, and let her experience *in imaginal* having sex with her normal partner. If the experience was a repeat of the former, unpleasant one, continue as follows:

> "And as you return to the present, here with me now, part of your mind will still be considering what it is that you know but don't know that you know, in relation to that former painful experience. And as soon as it becomes available to your conscious mind, you will become aware of it, and from that moment on you will be able to respond normally and without any further painful vaginal spasms in the future."

It might take hours, days or weeks for the deeply hidden information to filter its way through to the client's awareness.

Changing the answer

A simple, but sometimes effective method is to ask the client to go deep inside herself and ask the question,

Why does your vagina keep saying no?"
Wait for an answer.

Then ask,

"What would happen if your vagina said yes?"

Questionnaire

Beliefs

1. do you have any strong religious beliefs?
2. do you have any strong religious beliefs about sex?
3. do you believe that a man should dominate sexually?
4. do you believe that it is a woman's duty to please her partner sexually?

Relationships

1. how would you describe your relationship with your partner?
2. has there been any time in the past when the relationship was
    a) satisfactory
    b) good
    c) really good
    d) perfect?

3. is there a part of your relationship that frightens you?
4. have you ever felt hostility towards your partner? Describe
5. has your partner at any time had any kind of sexual disorder?

Sexual Relationships

1. are there any aspects of sex that you find pleasurable?
2. do you mind being touched by your partner?
3. do you place any limitations on your partner (,.e. certain parts of the body he may not touch)?
4. does your partner place any limitations on you?
5. is your partner very demanding sexually?
6. do you sometimes/often find yourself compelled to enter into sex without your approval?
7. what would happen if you refused?
8. has your partner tried means other than intercourse to bring sexual pleasure to you? Describe
9. have you tried means other than intercourse to bring sexual pleasure to your partner? Describe

Upbringing

1. were you brought up strictly?
2. what was your mother's attitude towards sex?
3. what was your father's attitude towards sex?
4. when you were a child, did anything happen to frighten you sexually?
5. how would you describe your relationship with your mother?
6. how would you describe your relationship with your father?
7. what sort of relationship did you have with brothers/sisters?

Body Image

1. what do you think of your hair? Style, texture, colour, etc?
2. how about your eyes?
3. nose. Are you satisfied with it? Would you like it changed in any way?
4. how about your mouth? Are you satisfied with it?
5. voice. How do you feel about your voice?
6. what about your arms?
7. how about your hands?
8. your overall figure. What do you think about it? Height, weight, etc.?

9. how about your breasts? Are they too big, too small, too saggy?

10. and the nipples. Are they too dark, too small, too big?

11. how about your stomach? How do you feel about your stomach?

12. and how about your hips?

13. genitals. How do you feel about your genitals?

14. do you ever feel that your vagina is too tight, too small?

15. what about your buttocks? Satisfied?

16. what about your thighs? How do you feel about your thighs?

17. legs?

18. feet? Satisfied or not satisfied with your feet?

19. how about your personality? How do you feel about that?

20. how do you feel about your partner's body? Are there any parts that frighten or disgust you? Describe

Outline of Dysfunctions

1. under what circumstances have you experienced an orgasm, if ever?

2. do you prefer masturbation to intercourse?

3. have you ever had a happy sex relationship other than with present partner?

4. at what point did you first experience vaginismus?
5. how does your partner generally respond to your discomfort? Does he understand and try to be gentle? Does he get angry or violent?

Chapter 2

Introduction to Sex Kinesiology – Male (SKM)

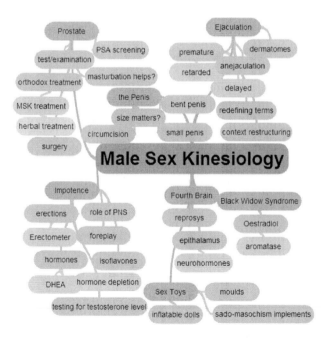

Male Impotence

Medomalacuphobia – the fear of losing an erection

Ithyphallophobia – the fear of seeing, thinking about,
or having an erect penis

Our sexuality should be amongst the greatest blessings that life has to offer. But sometimes difficulties arise from our desire to express ourselves sexually.

Obtaining accurate information about human sexuality used to be very limited. When I practised as a sexologist in the UK in the early 70s, I was one of only 5 professional sexologists in the country. 30-odd years ago. Now there are hundreds.

Treatment for the problems has changed very little over the years. The same problems exist, but so do the same treatments. And nearly of them are lengthy – if they work at all.

The changing point for me was when I began to learn about kinesiology. *Sex Kinesiology*, of course, didn't exist in those days, and I only developed it as I became more proficient in muscle-testing and could see the enormous potential it offered.

Let's take a brief look at the history of sexology – in the West. In the Orient, of course, it had been discussed for many centuries.

- Before Freud, the normal and natural goal of sexual desire was reproduction. He saw it as individual gratification.
- Krafft-Ebbing then introduced a concept of perversity, which Havelock Ellis called a 'new understanding' of sex
- Oscar Wilde, and his trial, raised homosexuality as a popular issue
- Virginia Woolf, in her writings, introduced the concept of free love and same sex love
- D.H Lawrence and Henry Miller introduced obscenity into writing, which led the way to just about 'anything goes' now

Male impotence, by which is meant difficulty or inability to attain and maintain an erection, is the most common of all male sexual dysfunctions. Although mainly psychogenic it can nevertheless be caused by a very wide range of other factors. It is said that most men experience impotence to some degree at some stage in their life.

Matter is not an aggregation of particles. It's a series of condensed spaces. Mass is condensed space. A piece of matter is as powerful as it can be made to expand its spaces.

If you put a piece of soft iron near a large enough magnet, in a few days the piece of iron will disappear. It's the same with cancer, which is a mass of irregular cells. If you expand the space between the cells, the tumour will break down and disappear.

The person with this problem, impotence, has a body that can't exude efficiently. A person is destroyed only by what he himself creates. And a release is something that lessens restrictions on an individual. I'll return to this shortly, and you'll see what I mean.

Penile erections, which are controlled by the Parasympathetic Nervous System, occur when the vascular reflex mechanism pumps blood into the cavernous sinuses of the penis, thereby enabling it to become firm or hard. Without at least some degree of erection, the penis is unable to penetrate the vagina to allow coitus to take place. The man's ability to feel passionate and aroused is not always sufficient to achieve erection.

Erectile dysfunction can be caused by some anatomical defect, e.g.
- a lesion of the Central Nervous System,

- or the posterior urethra;

Functional impotence, which is a general disruption of bodily functioning, can be due to

- spinal disease,
- drug over-use,
- certain endocrinopathies,
- aging,
- excessive fatigue, etc.;
- and Psychogenic causes can be
- anxiety
- negative attitudes to the opposite sex
- maladaptive patterns
- fear of being caught or disturbed, etc.

Most sexologists talk about

Primary Impotence as being where a male has never been able to achieve coitus,

Secondary Impotence where he has been successful on at least one occasion, and

Facultative Impotence where a male may have an erection with some partners and not with others.

Erection may occur during foreplay, then be lost on attempting, or soon after, penetration; may have an erection while clothed, but lost on being exposed to view; may erect for the purpose of masturbation or fellatio, but not for intercourse.

Some men are hypersensitive and therefore require very little stimulation, while others are hyposensitive and require a great deal of stimulation. Still others are only able to erect in special circumstances, e.g. fetishists, sadomasochists, paedophiliacs, etc. What are generally called 'Sexual Deviations', but what I prefer to call 'Sexual Variations', and are the subject of a separate Sex Kinesiology Special Health Report.

One of the inevitable side-effects of erectile dysfunction is the blow to a man's self-esteem, commonly resulting in *secondary depression.* So it becomes necessary to establish early on, during the interview, whether a client's primary depression is creating the sexual impotence, or whether the impotence is causing a secondary depression. The way this is established is to determine which came first. In the case of primary depression it becomes necessary to deal with the depression before attempting to deal with the impotence.

There are exceptional cases of hormonal imbalance which can affect erection, e.g. Klinefelter's syndrome, but since these require measurements of FSH, LH and Prolactin in serum and urine, this really comes outside the scope of the present Health Report. Hormone imbalance is more likely to affect female sexuality than male.

Organic causes of impotence are not common, except that any condition which can disturb the natural flow of blood to the penis or nerve supply may have an effect. Some complications of fractures to the pelvis, which involve both blood vessels and nerves, can disturb erection. And because erection commences with stimulation of the parasympathetic nerves of the pelvis, it can be disturbed by surgical removal of tissues of the rectum, bladder or prostate.

Other medical causes include:

- pulmonary disease
- renal disease
- cardiac disease
- many degenerative diseases
- malignancies
- some infections in the pelvic region
- any condition which may cause irritation during the sexual response
- hypertension

There are a number of drugs which tend to block the parasynpathetic nerves and thus interfere with erection, especially those prescribed for hypertension, and some for depression. These are listed in the questionnaire form, below.

Neurologic disorders affecting erection can result from severe malnutrition and vitamin deficiency, spina bifida, multiple sclerosis, herniated discs, etc. And some vascular diseases such as the Leriche syndrome (thrombotic obstruction of the aortic bifurcation), thrombosis of veins or arteries of the penis, leukaemia, sickle cell disorders, etc. Obviously, medical disorders such as any of these can only be dealt with by a medically qualified person.

Environmental causes, e.g. unemployment, unsatisfactory marriage or other relationship, heavy smoking, excessive intake of alcohol or some other drug, can all contribute dramatically to erectile dysfunction, as can faulty techniques due to ignorance, excessive preoccupation with the quality of performance, over-concern for partner, or even fear of failure.

Because erectile dysfunction (sensory response) is so different in character to ejaculatory dysfunction (motor response), so our approach to treatment needs to be different.

Close observation should be made of breathing (shallow, abdominal, etc.) and muscular rigidity (way client holds shoulders, stands or sits erectly, moves stiffly or jerkily). It is sometimes necessary to spend one or more sessions correcting breathing or postural abnormalities that are preventing client from relaxing.

Medical or physical causes need to be dealt with by a suitably qualified practitioner, either self or passed on. There are some instances where counselling is preferable to other forms of therapy, at least initially.

Sometimes a client needs to be made aware that satisfactory sex frequently – not always – needs an element of feeling, and it should not necessarily be regarded as a mechanical act of release, though there are occasions where that is what it's used for.

This applies particularly where a client's Primary Sensory Perception is kinaesthetic (his sense of touch and feeling are more developed than other senses, i.e. visual, auditory, etc.). He might need to know that masturbation is OK, even for adults. Childhood learning might have led him to believe it was bad, dirty, childish, harmful, and so on. Such early beliefs may go on to prevent him from erecting all through adult life, or until such time as a therapeutic remedy is installed.

Loss of erection is a phase surprisingly common in the 20s and 40 plus years. Depending on the psychological response, the phase may be temporary or longer lasting. In the 20s most males would consider themselves in their sexual prime, and to suddenly encounter loss of erection on a number of occasions can be devastating. Sometimes, merely knowing that this phase is not uncommon, and is likely to pass, can be sufficient to help the client overcome the phase.

Then, too, there is the question of *expected performances*. Some males feel their partner's expectation of them are higher than they are able to satisfy, and sexual anxiety can become acute or even chronic. Counselling is often an adequate way of dealing with that sort of problem, and it is sometimes helpful if partner is able to attend. Similarly, if client has failure expectancy, thereby creating a panic.

And, of course, the problem might stem from totally inadequate sexual foreplay. There are many females who refuse to touch or handle their partner's penis, and he might therefore be deprived of sufficient stimulation. So sexual techniques will have to be learned or improved and, again, it is often useful if partner agrees to attend.

Treatments

To return to what I was saying earlier, what have we got?

1. a person can't erect. Test a muscle, which should test weak.

2. in terms of what I was saying, this means he cannot condense space
3. he has created this condition himself
4. he wants to release the restriction he has placed on himself.

In order to do this he has to create something new. Let him create:

- 3 different places he'd like to be, and go there (in his mind, of course)
- put barriers that prevent him from going back*
- then put 3 different naked bodies there
- put ridiculous clothing on these bodies
- then let him see himself limp and flaccid
- then let him create an enormous erection
- test a muscle, which should now be strong

    *once we start erecting barriers we soon begin to think there are more barriers than there are

Here's something else, on the same theme:

A blind man knows he can't defend his body, so he fixes his body so that nobody will want it.

In a way, fixing your penis so it won't erect is a way of giving up ownership. But an inerection is only a symbol. It won't work properly, but it's still there. Like a car. You can sell a car and lose title to your ownership of it. But the car still exists. The certificate of ownership is a symbol.

An erection is a symbol. A symbol of manhood. Young men often brag about their ability to erect. To lose that is to lose a symbol. When you lose a symbol, you create a need to replace it with another symbol.

Technique

- give 3 things you have
- give 3 things somebody else has
- give 3 things others have for you
- give 3 things you have for another
- give 3 things you don't have (run in brackets, i.e. as if you're watching on TV)
- give 3 things you have deeds of title to (run in brackets)
- give 3 things you don't have deeds of title to (run in brackets)
- give 3 kinds of sex you don't object to

Symptom Utilisation

Sometimes a therapist is reluctant to use the simplest method because it seems *too* simple. Milton Erickson was the master of simplicity and I have adapted his *symptom utilisation* technique to impotency in the following manner (having the client fully relaxed and breathing deeply):

"What a pleasant change it makes to find a male who isn't bragging about how virile he is. I get so many patients coming to see me who have the complete opposite to your problem. And it seems that every time you pick up a newspaper the news seems to be hogged by men working off their excessive sex needs in one way or another.

"The television too seems preoccupied with the sexual needs of men. The problem I often have is that the treatment of their problems often takes quite a long time, whereas the occasional male that I get with your sort of problem invariably overcomes it so quickly that I find myself back with the other kind of problem all too soon. Anyway, you don't want to be bothered by that. Now, would you like to do this with your eyes open or closed?"

From that point, the client has become predisposed towards treatment in two ways. He believes his problem to be relatively minor, thus creating relief as well as strengthening his belief system in therapy; secondly, by asking him whether he wants to do it with his eyes open or closed, whichever he answers is a predisposition towards entering into treatment from which he expects to emerge favourably changed.

Restructuring

Restructuring means making a contract with yourself. Sometimes there is a need to retain an element of a neurosis and when this is the case it is preferable if the presenting problem, impotence in this case, can be ameliorated in such a way that a less-handicapping symptom can be substituted. I have used this technique in the following ways:

- client makes a contract with himself only to experience erectile dysfunction upon waking, or between 2-4 pm, only on a Sunday morning
- only when partner is an aborigine, Eskimo, or Polynesian (or any partner he is *unlikely* to ever encounter)
- only with a white-haired partner
- only with a partner over 1.80 cm

The options are without limit, and one can select situations which are not likely to occur in real life. The knowledge that the client can hang on to his symptom is his only requirement.

Metamorphosis

When we know from the questionnaire that a client has previously been virile at some earlier stage, we can begin to develop the idea of regressing him to that time, but in a way much different to normal regression therapy.

First we have to know something of the details of a particular occasion which he found erotic and in which he experienced no erectile difficulties.

Then we ask him to close his eyes and visualise a cinema screen, or television screen. If he can't visualise that, ask him to imagine that he is looking at one. Then we re-run a film of that erotic event that we already know about, in which the client sees himself experiencing what he already knows he has accomplished . So the remembrance is real, not fantasy, and can be reinforced by doing a second re-run, emphasising that what he has accomplished in the past he is capable of repeating.

This same technique can be used even when a client cannot recall a time in his life when he was capable of getting a full erection, by running a film in which he watches an idol (this can be someone he knows, or a film star, or whoever) perform how he would like to be able to perform himself. This can be repeated, and client can then be asked to stand in for his idol, and film is re-run again, this time with client playing the lead role.

If this is successful, and client can actually see himself getting an erection a new film can be made with client and his normal partner – if he has one, or fantasy partner if he hasn't. In the making of this film, he is asked to give a narration as he goes along, so therapist can keep check on what is happening. He is encouraged to see himself being completely successful.

Epithalamus

(This section should only be carried out by an experienced kinesiologist)

Is there a master centre that is responsible for sexual mechanics? There is, though not many people know about it. It's called the **epithalamus**, which includes the pineal gland, habenula and stria terminalis. The latter two belong to the limbic system – which we already know involves the hypothalamus.

The pineal gland produces a hormone called *melatonin*, which has a hitherto obscure relationship to the gonads. What we know is:

- melatonin regulates the production of all sex hormones, male and female
- melatonin regulates the circadian cycles in the human (through a dominating influence over *theta wave* activity), which in themselves have a powerful influence over the reproductive organs.

Melatonin is produced from serotonin, which requires the presence of tryptophan. We can check this amino acid out by going to St 45 (toe 2, lateral aspect) and muscle-testing. Because melatonin is derived by a two-step transformation of serotinin, to go to St 45 will in itself only give us information about serotonin. To get the additional information, we need to 2-point (touch both points simultaneously while muscle-testing) St 45 with the pineal gland itself. If this makes a strong muscle go weak it confirms the connection.

To correct, tap St 45 25 times while rotating pineal point about 10 times. As usual, retest to see if you have accomplished anything worthwhile.

Habenacular Nucleus

lies above and beside the pineal gland on each side. It communicates with the midbrain and is able to influence sex hormone production either by stimulating or inhibiting those hormones produced in the hypothalamus.

Stria terminalis

is a long strand of white matter, that influences the fibres that supply the nuclei of the brain stem. This area has the highest concentration of *opiate receptors* and is a major influence on mood and relaxation, both of which affect sex hormone production.

QUESTIONNAIRE

Body Image

1. What do you think of your hair? Style, texture, colour, etc?
2. How about your eyes?
3. Nose. Are you satisfied with it? Would you like it changed in any way?
4. How about the mouth? Are you satisfied with it?
5. Voice. How do you feel about your voice?
6. What about your arms? Do you have any tattoos or blemishes that embarrass you?

7. How about your hands?
8. Your overall figure? What do think of it? Height, weight, etc.?
9. What about your genitals? Are you satisfied with them?
10. Has a partner ever chided you on your genitals in any way?
11. What about your legs? Satisfied?
12. How about your feet?
13. How do you feel about your personality?
14. Do you ever compare your own penis with those of other men?
15. Do you feel comfortable in a public urinal?
16. Has a partner ever compared your penis to other men's?

Erections

1. Do you sometimes/frequently find an erection on waking up in the morning?
2. Do you ever awaken at night with an erection?
3. Are you able to achieve a full erection at any time?
4. Are you able to achieve a partial erection at any time? Describe.
5. Were you ever able to achieve a full erection? When? Under what circumstances?

6. Did you indulge in mutual masturbation with other boys?

7. Do you maintain an erection until (a) the point of penetration (b) after penetration (c) during actual intercourse?

Social Habits

1. Do you drink alcohol (in any form) heavily, moderately, not at all?

2. Do you occasionally smoke marijuana or any other similar?

3. Do you, or have you in the past, taken any harder drugs?

4. Are you satisfied with your social life?

5. Are you physically attracted to your partner?

6. Do you find others more attractive than your partner?

Masturbation

1. How often do you masturbate? If not now, when stopped?

2. Are you able to achieve full erection/partial erection during (a) self masturbation (b) masturbation by partner

3. Are you able to achieve erection up to ejaculation?

4. Of not, were you ever able to?
5. What form of masturbatory stimulation do you normally use?
6. Do you prefer masturbation to intercourse?

Medical

(1) Have you ever had any surgery? Describe.
(2) Have you ever had pain in lower back? Describe.
(3) Have you ever had, or do you have now, diabetes?
(4) Do you ever get any irritation in the genital area?
(5) Have you, or do you now, suffer from high blood pressure?
(6) Have you had any prescribed medication during the last six months?

(Note any of the following drugs:

Harmonyl	Enduronyl
Aldomet	Hydromet
Dopamet	Eutonyl
Hypovase	Salupres
Seominal	Marsilid
Tryptizol	Nardil
Sinequan	Concordin
Celtiprin	Pro-Banthine

Petrolinium   Methanthiline

Bromide   Propantheline

Hexamethonium   Clonidine

Mecamyalamine   Methyldopa

Amitryptiline   Antiepileptics

Antipsychotics   Beta   blockers

Antihypertensives

Sex Drive

1. Would you describe your sex drive as average, low, high, excessive?
2. What sort of things turn you on?
3. What sort of things turn you off?
4. Do you sometimes find it hard to concentrate on sex when you're having it?
5. Are you easily distracted by other thoughts when you are having sex?
6. Do you sometimes think of any other person when you're having sex?

Sexual Foreplay

1. Do you like lots of foreplay, or very little foreplay?
2. Who is the dominating partner during foreplay?

3. Does your partner ever remind you of someone else during lovemaking? Who?

4. Does your partner give you adequate stimulation during foreplay?

5. Are you able to discuss sex openly with your partner during foreplay? Are you able to say what you like and what you don't like?

6. Do you look forward to actual intercourse?

7. Do you ever fear you will fail to satisfy your partner?

8. If so, at what point does that fear begin?

Contraception

1. Do you or your partner usually use any form of contraception? If so, what type?

2. Are you or your partner concerned about possible pregnancy?

3. Have you, or have you ever had, any form of sexually transmitted disease? Specify.

4. Has your partner ever had an abortion/miscarriage?

Sexual Techniques

Describe a typical lovemaking session with your partner, starting at the very beginning, that is, at whose suggestion, time of day, place, how you or your partner normally begin, form of stimulation, and so on.

Sexual Ideals

2. Do you believe it is important for your partner to have enjoyment of sex as well as yourself?
3. Do you try to achieve simultaneous orgasm with your partner?
4. Do you consider it important that your partner has an orgasm?
5. Do you consider it important that you have an orgasm?
6. Do you talk during sex?
7. Do you have sex in the dark or in the light?
8. Describe your idea of perfect sex. Specify with whom it would be.

Programme for Optimal Sex Function

First step is to stop smoking. Nicotine is a strong vasoconstrictor with prolonged effect, and what you need for this problem is vasodilation.

Other things to avoid are:

- coffee, and anything else that contains caffeine (vasoconstrictor), including coca cola, and most soft drinks (esp. orange drink)

- theobromine, found in tea and chocolate
- Things to have:
- nuts
- vitamin E
- arginine
- zinc
- eggs

*   *   *

We can't leave the subject of impotence without mention of the role of eunuchs. The position of the eunuch in the power game was most interesting. The most renowned Chinese eunuch of all time was Admiral *Cheng Ho*, who led an expedition to the African coast in 1405 AD, the longest recorded expedition up to that period.

The status of the eunuch, because of the part he played in the most intimate affairs of men and women, gave him considerable influence where emperors and princes were most vulnerable. He had the perceptions of both sexes, to be suited to the special tasks, because he could appreciate the rational outlook of men, yet by the nature of his neutered physiology had the ability to understand female psychology.

His power in the court was achieved by the single-minded personal ambition of one suffering a deep bitterness and inferiority, on account of his deprivation. Because of this, all eunuchs realised that they had to be united with each other in order to advance themselves. They, therefore, formed a very powerful and ruthless clique. This cabal often formed the real power behind the throne and on many occasions carried out successful coups.

The psychologically traumatic nature of the castration itself and the different degrees of castration have been described by *Carter Stent*, a prolific writer on Chinese court life, manners and customs and first published in the *Journal of the Royal Asiatic Society* (North China Branch, 1877).

According to Stent, the castration operation is performed in the following steps. White cotton bandages are bound tightly around the lower part of the abdomen and the upper parts of both thighs, to minimise the haemorrhage. The genitalia are then bathed three times with hot peppered water. The subject (future eunuch) is now placed in a reclining position. When the parts have been sufficiently bathed they are cut off as closely as possible to the body with a small, curved sickle-shaped knife.

After the emasculation the wound is covered with six layers of rice paper saturated in ice water and is carefully bandaged tightly. After the wound is dressed, the eunuch is made to ambulate about the room, supported by two 'knifers' (surgeons) for two or three hours, after which he is allowed to rest. The eunuch is not allowed to drink anything for five days, during which time he often undergoes severe suffering from the impossibility of voiding urine. At the end of five days, the bandages are removed, whereupon the sufferer obtains some relief. If healing has satisfactorily taken place, he is considered out of danger and congratulated. Presents are showered on him. But if the unfortunate victim cannot void urine, he is doomed to a slow, uraemic death, as the urinary passages have become constricted.

There were three surgical forms of castration:

1. total excision
2. excision of the penis only
3. excision of both testicles

with total loss (*hsing ch'en*), once the wound had healed a metal, bamboo or straw tube was inserted into the urethra. Eunuchs retaining their testicles, frequently experienced unquenchable sexual desire, but were unable to perform. This was the unkindest cut of all.

This practice was continued until the fall of the Imperial Court in 1911.

*   *   *

A word of consolation if you're still worried about impotence: 73% of males are still naturally potent at the age of 70.

EJACULATION DYSFUNCTIONS

There is some difficulty in defining ejaculation dysfunctions because there is no common agreement between sexologists.

Some say that *premature ejaculation*

1. must precede intromission
2. if within 10 seconds of intromission
3. if within 1 minute of intromission

Masters & Johnson say it is premature if female does not achieve orgasm at least 50% of occasions when intercourse takes place. This does not allow for those cases where female orgasmic difficulties are present as a separate issue, so it is not a good definition.

My own definition is that premature ejaculation occurs when both partners regard it as a problem <u>providing</u> the female has been adequately stimulated prior to intromission, and is normally capable of achieving orgasm.

Retarded ejaculation occurs when a man cannot ejaculate intra-vaginally, sometimes termed *ejaculatory incompetence.*

Both premature and retarded ejaculation have been broken down, but I will give my own definitions rather than a whole list of others in order to avoid confusion:

- *Primary premature* – when satisfactory ejaculation during intercourse has never been achieved
- *Secondary premature* – when satisfactory ejaculation during intercourse has been achieved in the past but is no longer achieved
- *Tertiary premature* – when satisfactory ejaculation can be achieved during intercourse

with some partners but not with others

- *Primary incompetence* – when ejaculation intra-vaginally has never taken place
- *Secondary incompetence* – when intra-vaginal ejaculation has taken place in the past but no longer is

We can determine the nature of the problem, its probable causes, and whether treatment can be offered, after we have completed the appropriate stage of the questionnaire.

First, though, let's establish some of the bases of ejaculatory dysfunction. Ejaculation is controlled by the Sympathetic Nervous System, so anything that interferes with that might affect the ability to ejaculate, for example, organic causes (damage to genitals and their nerve supply, spinal injury, urethritis, prostatitis, etc.), drugs affecting sympathetic nervous functions.

Ejaculation consists of two stages:

1. when the seminal fluid enters the urethra ready for discharge, and
2. the discharge itself, which is the result of vigorous contractions of the muscles at the base of the penis.

The period immediately following ejaculation

is called the 'refractory' period, during which no further ejaculation can take place. This varies considerably between individuals. The Center for Marital and Sexual Studies in Long Beach, California recorded one male who had 16 ejaculations in one hour.

Taoist tradition tells us ...

> "A young and strongly built man can afford to ejaculate twice daily, but thin ones only once. A strong man of about 30 years of age can afford to do so once daily, whereas a weak man the same age should only do so once every two days. A strong man of 40 years of age can ejaculate once every three days, but a weak man this age should only do so once every four days. Strong men of 50 can safely do so every five days, whereas a weak man of fifty needs a rest of ten days. Strong men of 60 may healthily ejaculate every ten days, but weak men of the same age need 20 days in between. A strong man of 70 can ejaculate once a month without harm, but a weak man that age should not ejaculate anymore.

About 100 years ago, Alice Stockham wrote a book entitled *Karezza: Ethics of Marriage*, in which she supported the teachings of many *Tantric* and *Taoist* masters in the practice of 'semen retention'. During *karezza* intercourse, ejaculation is delayed indefinitely. It became popular in New York State towards the end of the 19th Century, and many articles appeared about that time enthusing about the technique. It was said that, once mastered, it enabled the male participant to have a dozen or more 'divine' orgasms without actually ejaculating.

As always, our first objective in treatment is to determine whether the problem is organic or psychogenic, or if it could be the results of drugs, etc. We should have the necessary information from the questionnaire, but if not we can always test using the Trauma Recall mode by putting head into extention or flexion and testing the muscle.

Organic Problems

Ejaculation is the propulsion of semen through the penile meatus. The neural pathways arise from the spinal levels T10 to L2, and travel through the sympathetic chain ganglia. It involves somatic efferent nerves through S2 to S4 and autonomic nerves T12 to L2.. In a healthy man, the *ejaculatory reflex* is initiated by sensory stimulation of the penis and by cerebral erotic input.

Ejaculation may fail to take place if the internal sphincter muscle fails to contact during orgasm. This could happen as a result of injury or damage sustained during an operation, or simply as a blocking effect on the sympathetic nerve supply as the result of some drugs.

In addition, there might be a failure of contraction of the seminal vesicles and *vasa deferentia* (ejaculatory duct) in which are stored the semen. In all of these cases, medical attention is required rather than any form of counselling or psychotherapy. The clues will come out in the questionnaire.

The ejaculate volume itself is normally 1.5-5 cc, and tends to decrease with age. The ejaculate consists of:

- ascorbic acid, inositol, B12
- blood group antigens
- calcium, magnesium, chlorine, sodium, potassium, nitrogen, phosphorus, zinc
- cholesterol, choline
- citric acid, lactic acid, pyruvic acid
- DNA
- fructose
- glutathione
- hyaluronidase
- purine, pyrimidine

- spermidine, spermine
- urea, uric acid

Psychogenic Problems

These are many and varied. A creaking bed, thin walls, a child sleeping in the same room, pain, anxieties, failure to satisfy, fear of pregnancy, lack of interest in partner, business or work worries, fear of discovery, and so on. You should be able to narrow these down from the questionnaire.

Many patients seeking help for ejaculatory disorders might already be taking prescribed drugs, i.e. tranquillisers, antidepressants, etc. changes brought about by these drugs are usually due to a lowering of anxiety leading to some kind of improvement in their sexual functioning rather than a change in their actual conditions.

Consequently, their subsequent sexual functioning may vary according to the continued use of these drugs, the diminishing effects of the drugs themselves as the body begins to adjust to them, and any change in the prescription. Combinations with other drugs may have an unforeseen effect also.

The Law of Reversed Effect

After Induction:

"You have become very concerned about your inability to delay ejaculation long enough to satisfy both yourself and your partner. But now, and in future, you might consider the possibility of being very, very concerned of *not being able to ejaculate*, regardless of how hard you try. The more you try, the more difficult it will become for you to ejaculate when you are having intercourse with your partner.

"You will not lose your erection, in fact your erection will grow *stronger and stronger*, but it will become *more and more difficult* for you to ejaculate *until your partner starts to come*.

"Your erection will grow *stronger and stronger* and you will be *enjoying* the intercourse more and more, but you will find it *impossible* to ejaculate until your partner has started to come.

"And then you will find something *unusual* happening to you. Once your partner has *started to come* you will find yourself *ready* to ejaculate. But this will be an orgasm so *powerful* that it will affect the *whole* of your body and mind. So *powerful* and so *exciting* that once it has happened to you will want it to be the same on every subsequent occasion that you have intercourse.

"So, on the very next occasion that you have intercourse, you are finding the following things happening without you consciously having to think about them happening. When you are starting to have sexual foreplay you are having no trouble at all getting a good erection. It doesn't matter whether your partner is playing with you or you are playing with your partner, you are having a good erection, but you are *not* ready to ejaculate. Similarly, when you first penetrate your partner's vagina, you have a good erection but you are *not* ready to ejaculate.

"In fact, as you proceed into the actual intercourse you are enjoying it *more and more*, and your erection is getting stronger and stronger. And as your erection grows stronger and stronger, and your enjoyment grows *greater and greater*, so you are finding your desire to ejaculate grows less because you are enjoying it so much you don't want it to end too quickly.

"In fact, it is becoming *impossible* to

ejaculate until you know that your partner is beginning to come. And when your partner begins to come, so you are finding yourself ready and able to ejaculate.

"And your ejaculation is so *powerful*, so *intense*, and so *exciting*, that it consumes the whole of your body and mind. And because this ejaculation is so powerful, and so perfectly co-ordinated with your partner's orgasm, you will want it to happen the same way on each subsequent occasion that you have intercourse. And because you *want* it to happen that way, so you are finding it *will* happen that way."

Redefining Terms

Sometimes it is possible to take words or thoughts or beliefs that a client has and redefine them in a different way, so that what had previously been a disadvantage can become an advantage.

Here is a technique I tried for a client who was an airline pilot and needed quick treatment because he had to go away for a long period in the Middle East. It worked instantly for him, and I have since tried it on very many other clients with a considerable success.

His definition of 'premature' was

ejaculating too quickly. So I *redefined* it in the following way:

> "How wonderful it is that you should be so anxious to satisfy your partner, and I can understand your eagerness to do so. But what has happened is that a part of your mind, deep, deep inside, out of your awareness, has mistaken your eagerness for mere speed, and has accordingly brought your own ejaculation earlier than you actually desired.
>
> "So now, just allowing your body and mind to drift gently until you reach that part of the mind responsible for your orgasm and ejaculation....... Drifting gently......... and just nod the head when you have made contact with that part of the mind........ (wait for indication). That's good. Now thank that part of your mind sincerely for having allowed you to have so many wonderful orgasms in the past, and thank it anticipation of all the fantastic orgasms you are to have in the future.
>
> "Thank it particularly *in anticipation* of it allowing you to *hold back your orgasm* a little longer so that your partner is equally able to achieve and enjoy her own orgasm

at the same time."

Context Restructuring

What we want to try and achieve is a context in which our client's present behaviour will be more appropriate.

In order to find out what that might be it is helpful to ask a few questions which appear to be totally unrelated to the problem. Like,

> "Do you find it difficult getting up in the morning?"
> "Are you late often getting to work?"
> "Are you ever late for appointments?"
> "Do you tend to leave paying debts to the very last moment?"
> "What about Income Tax, or bank overdrafts?"

The object is to keep asking innocuous questions like this until you have at least one or two areas where the client is late.

Then ask him to sit back and relax, take a few deep breaths, and go deep inside.

> "And I want you to think what premature ejaculation really means? It means being

early. And by being early with your ejaculation you are disappointing yourself and your partner.

"Now there are times when being early is a wonderful thing, but in respect of orgasms, being early is not a good thing. So I think it would be a good idea if you can find a suitable context where being early would be satisfying to you.

"Say, arriving at work early instead of being late. Would that be preferable?" (Wait for an affirmative indication). Okay. So try and visualise yourself arriving early for work. See the expression of pleasure on your own face as you do so.

"And on some other occasions, particularly when you are approaching orgasm with your partner, it can be so much more pleasurable for both of you, if you are 'late'. Perhaps you can visualise that."

Restore Systems Therapy

This is the wonderful technique that Microsoft uses with its new XP programme, which they call *Restore Systems*. We can apply it to humans by taking them back to a time (in their mind, because it won't be in real time) before they experienced the problem.

Sit the person down quietly, and when he is suitably relaxed ask him to go back in time to a point when the problem they have first started.

Test the muscle to see that they have arrived there. Muscle should be weak. Then ask them to go back one day before the problem first appeared. Test muscle. Should be strong. If it is weak, proceed as follows:

1. Ask client to think of problem while you test the muscle. If the muscle is still weak, put the head into *flexion* and retest. If the muscle is now strong indicates that the problem is psychogenic.
2. If muscle is still weak, put head into *extension* and retest. If muscle is now strong indicates that problem is organic.
3. If the problem is psychogenic, then treat as in Trauma Recall, that is, by putting head into flexion 3 times while client thinks of problem.
4. If the problem is organic, you will have to investigate the whole range of organic possibilities and eliminate them in turn until you find the influential core. Until you know

that that is, we cannot say how to treat.

If, on the initial test above, the muscle tests strong, then we can anchor that 2 or 3 times on the arm, then take client forward one day (to the time when problem began) and retest. Stimulate anchors repeatedly while client thinks about the problem. After about 1-2 minutes of this, retest muscle while client thinks of problem. If muscle is strong, indicates that anchoring has been effective.

Bring client back to present time and retest muscle. Should be strong.

Autonomic Therapy

While the process of erections is governed by the parasympathetic nervous system (PNS), the process of ejaculation is controlled by the sympathetic nervous system (SNS).

It is possible with the following SK technique to **retrain** the SNS responses to sexual stimulation. The orgasmic and ejaculation circuits centre in the spinal cord from T10-L2. There is a secondary major ejaculatory area in the pelvic cavity between the anus and the coccyx, which is the reason why some men and women enjoy anal sex so much.

What we do is test the spinal points T10-L2 and note any causing a weak muscle, but we treat the *dermatone point* as shown on the Scranton chart, either clockwise to stimulate (when there is retarded ejaculation or counter-clockwise where there is premature ejaculation. Then go back to the spinal point which went weak and retest.

The SK Qi Gong Technique

Men can achieve ejaculation control by shifting the nervous response circuits from the urethra-prostate nerves to the anal-tailbone nerves.

Exerting an inhaling (qi) pressure against the bladder is to turn on the bladder's sensory-parasympathetic nervous system circuits for overriding the prostate's sensory-sympathetic (ejaculation and orgasmic circuits). So does contracting the coccygeal muscle.

The centre of the front bladder is the location of the low body qi concentrative point (called Dan-Tien) between Ren 3 and Ren 4 (the Conception Vessel. Ren 1 (the Master of Yang qi) is the first point point of the Ren channel.

During this Qi Gong Breathing Exercise, the bladder's parasympathetic nerves discharge bioelectric flow into the Ren channel, and when you're contracting the coccygeal muscle, the bioelectric flow moves across the anus from Ren 1 (between the anus and scrotum, near the prostate) to Du 1, where the bioelectric energy partially flows in the Du (Governing) channel and partially feeds the sensory nerves around the coccyx (the sensory-parasympathetic circuits sacral nerves S1-S5 and Coccygeal nerve).

Then the bioelectric current in the sensory nerves is split into two parts in the interneuron switches/splitters inside S1-S5 and CO. A large part of energy is coupled into the spinal cord nerves/CNS to the brain's cerebral cortex (sensory and then motor areas for response). The rest of the bioelectric energy is reflected back to the genital area through the S1-S5 and CO parasympathetic motor nerves that drive the erection and engorgement blood pressures from the pubis/penis/groins to the coccyx.

If you contract the muscles of the *Urogenital Triangle* (the ischiocavernosus muscle, bulbospongiosus m, and the superior transverse perineal m) the energy due to sexual stimulation and muscle contraction (testosterone burning) will turn to the sensory-sympathetic nervous circuits (orgasmic/ejaculation) circuits between the urethral/prostate (or urethral/vagina) nerves and T10-L2 spinal cord interneuron switches/splitters.

<u>That means you activate the orgasmic/ejaculation circuits</u>. To prolong sex, you have to let the ejaculation circuits have a nap for a while.

To do this, you contract the coccygeal muscle during in breath and relax during out-breath for at least 3 complete cycles.

Then retest muscle to see if you have accomplished anything.

Guilt Removal

Sometimes, premature ejaculation is a direct result of feelings of guilt, or hostility towards partner, or memories of the past. There is a simple technique for dealing with these or any similar causes:

After induction:

> "And because you are now so deeply relaxed you are able to deal with any problem without experiencing any anxiety, stress or tension. And I would like you to imagine a glass case in front of you. I might be quite large, or whatever size you prefer. It is suspended, right in front of your eyes
>
> "What I would like you to do now is simply to put all your feelings of guilt (or hostility, or whatever) inside that glass case. And you can notice that your guilt, inside

that glass case, has got a colour. A very clear, distinct, strong colour. What colour is your guilt?" (Wait for answer)

"That's good. And now a very remarkable thing is happening. Even as you are looking at the contents of your glass case a white light is entering the case, enveloping all the contents in this bright, pure, cleansing light. Can you see the colour .... (whatever colour the client gave) beginning to change to white? (Wait for answer)

"And now another remarkable thing is happening. As the purifying white light is completely enveloping the glass case and its contents, you are noticing that the glass case is becoming empty. The colour that you saw inside (dissociating problem from colour now) has completely disappeared.

"And the wonderful thing is that it is as if a great weight has been lifted off you. You are beginning to feel the relief even now as I am talking to you. And all due to the fact that the colour you saw has completely gone ...."

Hypnotic States

Over the years, I have used hypnosis as a method of uncovering very many *difficult* cases of ejaculatory dysfunction. From time to time a therapist encounters a really stubborn case that does not respond to any of a whole range of treatments. In such a case, I tend to suspect a traumatic event that happened earlier in life. Here is a selection of such cases, with edited excerpts of their experience under hypnosis, to exemplify an underlying cause.

Case 1: *a 28-year-old father of two boys, separated 18 months as a result of his premature ejaculation problem:*

> "I am lying in the sun on our lawn. Mum and dad have gone out shopping. Rover is flopped out on the grass next to me ... his tongue is lolling and he is panting heavily. I ought to go and get him a bowl of water but I feel too tired and sleepy. I strip down to my underpants and lie with an arm cradled across my eyes, blotting out the harsh glare. I seem to doze off ... Seem to be floating ... looking down into a room, like I'm floating up against the ceiling ... looking down into the bedroom ... man is lying on bed, no clothes on ... his penis is large and is sticking out of a bush of hair ... a hand

appears and takes hold of the penis … it grows very hard and thick, like a tree stump … my heart is pounding, I'm afraid he will look up and see me watching him from above the bed … the hand is moving up and down the length of his penis, then I realise the hand doesn't belong to him … his arms are folded behind his head, but I can't see his face … I hear a voice, a woman's voice, 'Hurry up and come, my arm's aching' … Can't take my eyes off the hand and the penis … very red, glistening, hand moving up and down faster and faster … I float down a bit lower, something makes me want to see a face … 'Hurry up, else I'm going' … it's the woman's voice again, she seems bored … I can see the man's mouth now, but not the face … it's smiling, opening up to reveal crooked, yellow teeth … 'Shut up and do your job,' it seems to say … the hand stops moving … 'I've told you, hurry up or I'm going,' the woman's voice says again … the hand starts moving up and down again … something bursts out of the end of the penis … it's coming straight up towards me … I try to get away, it's as if I've been caught spying on them … the stuff catches me right in the belly, like I've been kicked by a horse ... it goes right through me, there's a gaping hole where my belly had been ... I start to fall ... falling, dropping like a stone ... wind screams through the hole in my belly ... I seem to land with a searing pain ... the huge penis has pierced through my belly, like a skewer ... thick, sticky fluid oozes all over me ... the woman is cackling like an old witch ... as the sticky, pungent goo floods into my eyes the last thing I see is the face of the man ... my father --- the woman's voice is still cackling 'I told you to come quickly'."

After effects: "I feel disgusted with my father. I don't ever want to be like that."

Post-abreactive discussion: Patient's age at time of dream was eleven. He has just been introduced to masturbation by schoolmate and told how babies come about. His first reaction was disbelief. He couldn't imagine that his father could do anything so *dirty*. Further experiments of masturbating with friend and alone always ended in the same way, with patient wanting to get it over as quickly as possible. Once problem had been identified with a 'dream', the patient felt reassured and the ejaculatory problem ended instantly.

Case 2: *A 22-year-old male student, attempted suicide on three occasions due to depression arising from ejaculatory disorders.*

> "I feel like a top, spinning round and round, turning, bobbing … there is pressure in my left side, like a fist pushing into me … my visual field is dark … dark and heavy, with a tiny red pin-prick of light in the centre … the left side of me feels heavier than the right … the red pin-prick has disappeared and everything is completely black now … vibration … I am jerking, dizzily … nothing makes any sense … how can I get through? I feel some tingling down my spine … a face leers at me through the dark … not a human face … a seal, or walrus, I don't know exactly … eyes piercing, tongue lashing out at me, like a snake's … God, it <u>is</u> a snake, lunging at me, spitting venom at me … my head is spinning, sweaty, throbbing, vibrating … I'm trying to run, but where to? I'm in a hole, wedged inside a hole … the snake's back, spitting at me, I can't get out of the hole … trapped!"

After-effects: Splitting headache, followed by willingness to co-operate in other treatments, which had previously been resisted.

Post-abreactive discussion: This regression had highlighted patient's obsession first with sex, and with difficulties in dealing with life's problems and pressures. The black void, the fear of being trapped were all symbolic of his fears of sex. His answer was to get out as quickly as possible, to run away, to escape, to *ejaculate* quickly. Further treatment of changing context, and helping to come to terms with the stresses of life, helped him overcome his ejaculatory dysfunction.

QUESTIONNAIRE

<u>Body Image</u>

1. What do you think about your hair? Style, texture, colour, etc.
2. How about your eyes?
3. Nose. Are you satisfied with it? Would you like it changed in any way?
4. How about your mouth? Are you satisfied with it?
5. Voice. How do you feel about your voice?

6. What about your arms?

7. How about your hands?

8. Your overall figure. What do you think about it? Height, weight, etc.

9. What about your genitals? Are you satisfied with them?

10. Has a partner ever chided you on your genitals in any way?

11. Have you ever compared genitals with any other male? As a child? As an adult?

12. Has any partner ever compared your genitals with that of other men?

13. What about your legs? Satisfied?

14. And how about your feet?

15. How do you feel about your personality?

Sex Drive

1. How would you describe your own sex drive: a) average; b) low; c) high d) excessively high/low

2. What sort of things turn you on?

3. What sort of things turn you off?

4. Do you sometimes find yourself having sex more out of duty than desire?

5. Do you sometimes find it hard to concentrate on sex when you're having it?

6. Can you remember how you first learned about

sex?

7. Do you think your sex drive is stronger/weaker than before?

Medical

1. Have you ever had any surgery? Specify.
2. Have you ever had any inflammation in the genital or anal area?
3. Have you ever had any massage or other treatment for such inflammation?
4. Have you ever had mumps?
5. Have you had, or do you still have, high or low blood pressure?
6. Have you had, or are you still having, any medication for hypertension: (note any of the following drugs: Esbatol Declinax   Ismelin Eutonyl (delayed ejaculation)   Anafrinil Pertofran   Tofranil   Berkomine Rogitine Aldomet   Dopamet Hydromet   Cozaar

Ejaculation

1. Are you ever able to achieve ejaculation during intercourse?
2. Do you ejaculate before entry? Always usually occasionally
3. How long after penetration does ejaculation

usually occur?

4. Were you ever able to achieve ejaculation during intercourse? When?

5. Do you have nocturnal ejaculation frequently occasionally?

6. Do you indulge in foreplay? Too much too little?

Masturbation

1. How often do you masturbate? If not now, when stopped?

2. At what age did you first masturbate?

3. Are you normally able to achieve ejaculation during masturbation?

4. How long, during masturbation, does ejaculation normally take?

5. What form of masturbatory stimulation do you normally use?

6. Does your partner masturbate you to ejaculation a) occasionally b) frequently c) never

7. Do you prefer masturbation to intercourse?

Intercourse

1. Where does sexual intercourse normally take place?

2. At any particular time of the day, normally?
3. Have you ever had intercourse in a situation where you have felt a) uncomfortable (e.g. In the back of a car); b)fearful of being caught (e.g. In public place, parents' home, etc.); c) with a prostitute (i.e. When there was a time pressure)
4. How do you rate intercourse on a scale of 0-10?
5. What is the highest value you have ever given it (from 0-10)?
6. When was that?
7. Do you ever have sex with anyone apart from your wife/present partner?
8. Do you have the same, or similar, problem then?

Contraception

1. Do you or your partner usually any form of contraception?
2. Do you, have you ever, used the rhythm method?
3. Are you or your partner concerned about possible pregnancy?
4. Has your partner (or any other partner) ever had an abortion or miscarriage?

Sex Ideals

1. What is your idea of perfect sex? Specify with whom it would be.
2. When should ejaculation take place during intercourse?
3. Is it important for your partner to have an orgasm simultaneously?
4. Are you concerned whether your partner has an orgasm at all?

Foreplay

1. Do you require a lot or very little tactile stimulation?
2. Do you object to too much foreplay?
3. Do you not object to but derive little pleasure from foreplay?
4. Do you find sexual foreplay actually displeasurable?
5. Do you prefer foreplay to intercourse?

Hormone Depletion Therapy

Over-masturbation or over-ejaculation by any means, can cause a depletion of neurochemicals in the brain, spine and local tissues. A deficiency of acetylcholine will cause the underproduction of the local relaxant hormone prostaglandin E-1, which helps relax the neurons for stretching and bending of ligaments, muscles and joints. You will feel muscular pulling pains in the body, especially in the low back, low abdomen and groin. You may also experience testicular and hernial pains too. It can also cause erectile dysfunction.

When you deplete the acetylcholine neurochemicals by seminal discharge, your liver and adrenal functions become partially deactivated. Your liver cannot supply sufficient enzymes for hormone and neurotransmitters (such as acetylcholine, dopamine and serotonin) production. And your adrenal glands cannot produce sufficient DHEA and androstenedione to power your brain's and testicular functions.

Regarding premature ejaculation, you have trained your sympathetic nerves to have a quick orgasm or ejaculation response to sexual stimulation. Your weak erection won't create a high blood pressure inside your penile shaft to compress the urethral/prostate nerves and block their sensing and communication.

With a weak erection, you frequently exercise your perineal muscles in order to revive your erection. In turn, it stimulates your bulbourethral glands to produce a lot of precum, which contains a lot of the ripening hormone prostaglandin E-2, which opens the ejaculation duct for semen emission, even without orgasmic contraction in the prostate and seminal vesicles and their adjacent muscles.

Generally, premature ejaculators can produce a lot of precum by a simple visual or auditory stimulation or even kissing, without touching the genitals. The precum production is stimulated by the sympathetic nervous function, but it can be down-modulated by the serotonin nervous function.

With a depletion of serotonin neuro-chemicals, you will suffer anxiety, stress, ADD, sleeping disorder, and emotional instability. Serotonin can help reduce conversion of dopamine to norepinephrine and epinephrine in the nervous system and adrenal medulla (and bloodstream).

Serotonin is converted to melatonin by the pineal gland during the dark, where melatonin brings your brain to deep sleep which helps your pituitary gland produce a lot of Human Growth Hormone to support your entire body functions.

Apart from over-ejaculation, a deficiency of serotonin can also be caused by a deficiency of the amino acid tryptophan. We can test for this in the usual way through kinesiology.

Chapter 3

Introduction to Sports Kinesiology – (SpK)

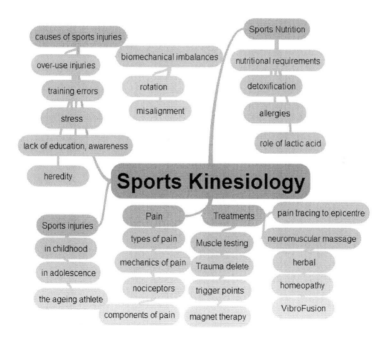

Sports Kinesiology has been developed by Harry Howell in response to the growing needs of practitioners to help deal with sports-related injuries, positive motivation, etc. It enables practitioners to establish a root problem quickly and to deal with the problem just as quickly. The complete course takes 2-3 years to complete, depending on the student's kinesiology skills.

The programme focuses on hypertonic (over-tight) muscles, releasing them through muscle activation techniques and Qi-gong breathing exercises. Also promotes the flow of Cerebro Spinal Fluid, improves body/mind integration and performance, as follows:

Ankle injuries	anxiety
Arthritis	bruises
Bursitis	carpal tunnel synd
Cold	collapse
Concussion	cramp
Exhaustion	fainting
Fatigue	fractures and sprains

Head injuries	heel injuries
Hip, pelvis and groin injuries	knee injuries
Ligament strain	lower back injuries
Lower leg injuries	stress fractures
Tarsal tunnel syndrome	tendinitis
Wounds, cuts	other injuries

General examination and treatment procedures

Meridian therapy

Stomatognathic system

Mental and emotional conditions

Respiratory adjustment

Orthopaedic conditions

Acupressure trigger points

Introduction to Homeopatia

Introduction to VibroFusion

Emotional stress release

The 14 channels and their related muscles

Coordination of Mind and Body

Causes of sports injuries

- Over-use injuries

    Warning signs

    Masking a major disorder

    Violation of Natural Law

- Training errors
- Biomechanical imbalances

    rotations

    misalignments

- Stress – Body, Mind, Spirit, Social and Environmental
- Lack of education and awareness – ignorance of body and social messages
- Mental factors – excess anger, grief, greed, etc.
- Heredity – bad genes resulting in increased or decreased needs

Nutrition

- An understanding of basic nutrition

- A nutrition body map – body pits that can be used for checking deficiencies
- How to use SpK to test for amino acid requirements
- Special nutritional needs for athletes
- Blood sugar and how it affects sports activities

Detoxification

- The organs of elimination
- The importance of effective eliminative processes
- Lactic acid and its role in the body
- Detoxification programmes

Homeopathy

- What it is and how it works
- The scope of homeopathy in sports
- Complex homeopathy for spots injuries

VibroFusion

- Dealing with pain

cramping

pain from acid conditions

pain from alkaline conditions

pain from self-made toxins, injury

- Pain where cold improves
- Pain where heat improves
- Pain where motion improves
- Pain where no motion improves
- Pain where touch improves
- Pain where no touch improves
- Suborbital, migraine, temporal headaches
- Intercostal neuralgia
- Large joint discomfort in knees, low back, elbows, shoulders
- Low back pain
- Small joint pain in fingers, toes

Allergies

- The nature of allergies and/or intolerances
- How they can affect sports activities
- How to test for allergies, using SpK

- How to treat allergies, using SpK

Acupressure

What it is and its uses for the sportsman

Acupressure pain relief points

Acupressure for:

- Arm injuries
- Inflammation of biceps tendon
- Tennis elbow
- Golfer's elbow
- Inflammation of forearm tendons
- Wrist injuries
- Carpal tunnel syndrome, and simple treatment
- Sprained thumb and fingers
- Spinal injury
- Thoracic spinal injuries
- Lumbar spine
- Trunk injuries
- Stitch
- Groin and hip injuries

- Abdominal sprain
- Thigh injuries
- Rectus femoris
- Hamstring
- Ligaments
- Cartilages
- Lower leg injuries
- Inflammation of Achilles tendon
- Leg cramp
- Ankle injuries
- Pain on sole of foot
- Pain on ball of foot
- Pain on bunion joint of foot

Chinese Qi Gong Techniques

- Bone marrow massage to strengthen bones
- The spine – to strengthen nerve supply to joints
- Joints
- Highly effective breathing exercise

Arthritis and Sports

- Rheumatoid arthritis
- Osteoarthritis
- Ankylosing spondylitis
- Rheumatism

Sports Injuries in Childhood and Adolescence

- Pain in the bones
- Pain and swellings at knee
- Pain in the growth plate in the heel
- Joint injuries
- In-toeing and out-toeing
- What children can do for weak feet
- Limping and pain at hip
- Hip and groin pain with awkward gait

The Ageing Athlete

- Running when you're older
- Idleness and ageing
- How and where ageing happens

Hand and Foot Acupressure and Electrical Treatments

- A complete microcosmic system of treating the whole body – without needles
- The use of magnet for sports injuries
- Electromagnetic therapy for faster healing and pain relief/control

WHAT IS PAIN?

How it Affects Body and Mind

Neck Pain – Cervical

The word pain is derived from Greek *ponos* and Latin *paean*. It is a sensation of hurt. It is the body's way of alerting us that something is wrong. Pain is, without doubt, the most distressing common experience, yet it has no precise definition. Also, there is no specific organ that we can associate with pain. We don't have a pain organ, although all organs can experience pain.

Pain has obvious sensory qualities, but it also has emotional and motivational properties. It is usually caused by intense noxious stimulation, yet it sometimes occurs spontaneously without apparent cause. It normally indicates physical injury, but it sometimes fails to occur when extensive areas of the body have been seriously injured. At other times it persists even after all the injured tissues have healed.

History of Pain and its Treatments

Man has been afflicted with pain since the beginning of evolution. As the records of every race are examined, one finds records of the omnipresence of pain. In every civilisation and in every culture, prayers, exorcisms and incantations are found which bear testimony to the dominance of pain.

It is natural, then, that since its beginning mankind should have been engaged in its quest to find ways of controlling and eliminating it. To the present day, we have managed to find some methods of eliminating some types of pain, or reducing it, or managing it. We have even developed some concepts that help us to understand it.

During the course of this section, I will show some of the giant strides that we can take to understand it more, to at least reduce most types of pain, and even to eliminate pain that has defied all other forms of treatment.

Probably the earliest attempts at managing pain included physical therapeutic methods, like rubbing or massage or exposure to cold water from streams and lakes, or using the heat of the sun and later that of fire. Pressure was also used to benumb the part to lessen pain.

When primitive man could not relieve his own suffering he called on the head of the family, very often a priestess or sorceress, or a medicine man. As the centuries rolled by, man's idea of the cause of pain underwent a change. With the arrival of Christianity, a new concept of pain relief based on divine healing through the laying on of hands and prayer – still very strong today.

In addition to prayer, priests employed natural remedies consisting mostly of medicinal herbs. The use of herbs came to us from ancient times, before recorded history. They had been used by primitive man, who had experimented with various plants as foods, discovering that some of them were helpful in relieving pain. Their use was gradually taken over first by the priest, then by the medicine man, and then by the early physicians.

We'll be discussing the merits of different foods, some of which can induce pain, others which can be helpful in reducing pain.

The use of analgesic drugs derived from plant life was prominent in all ancient cultures, using such plants as the poppy, hemp and henbane. The hundreds of years of the Middle Ages contributed comparatively little to man's knowledge of alleviating pain. The Renaissance engendered a great scientific leap that made many remarkable advances in science, particularly in chemistry and physics. But it hardly made any contribution to the relief of pain.

The new era of analgesia began in 1772 with Priestley's discovery of *nitrous oxide*. This period was culminated by the first public demonstration of surgical anaesthesia at the Massachusetts General Hospital in Boston in 1846, by Morton. In 1817 Frederick Sertuner has published his paper naming the new alkaloid of opium after Morpheus, the Greek god of dreams. The importance of getting pure crystalline drugs from previous crude and uncertain mixtures was eventually realised, and very soon after other opium alkaloids were isolated.

The chance findings of the pain relieving properties of Willow bark by an 18th Century English village priest named Stone was one of the beginnings of finding better analgesics. Acetylsalicylic acid, known as aspirin, is still widely used, often as a first choice pain remover.

Synthetic chemistry began to produce narcotic analgesic compounds that proved to be equal, if not superior, to the natural opiates. Inhalation analgesia and anaesthesia was being introduced into surgical practice, and another method was being initiated in France, the USA, Ireland and Scotland: the introduction of the metallic hollow needle in 1843 and the syringe in 1853.

The isolation of cocaine in 1855 was a milestone in the conquest of pain. Many primitive people of South

America, Africa and Asia were already aware of the use of coca leaves for the relief of pain of the larynx and pharynx.

The 19th Century produced yet another great advance in the conquest of pain by surgical methods. As soon as it became possible to operate without fear of infection a number of surgeons throughout the world independently began to attack the age-old problem of pain by permanent interruption of its neural pathways.

After the discovery of X-ray by Roentgen, deep penetrating roentgen rays were employed in the treatment of severe and persistent pain. The place of X-ray therapy in the treatment of pain of carcinogenic origin is still in extensive use.

The entire concept of the mechanism of the feeling of pain has changed recently. Melzack and Wall discovered the Gate Control Theory of Pain. Basically, the theory of pain proposes that a neural mechanism in the dorsal horn of the spine acts like a gate that can increase or decrease the flow of nerve impulses from peripheral fibres to the Central Nervous System (CNS). This theory coincides with the acupuncture treatment of pain.

In 1973, Snyder and Pert found out during their researches on drug addiction that there are some clusters of cells in the brain that attract narcotic drugs. They termed these cells as *opiate receptors*. The cells were used by the body to attract natural enkephalins that bring relief of pain.

The latter stages of the 20th Century saw developments taking place within Alternative Medicine in very interesting, novel, and effective ways. We'll be charting these new concepts throughout this section.

Of course, I could have given a more account of the history of pain, like this:

> "Doctor, I have an ear ache."
> 2000 B.C. – "Here, eat this root."
> 1000 A.D. – "That root is heathen, say this prayer."
> 1850 A.D. – "That prayer is superstition, drink this potion."
> 1940 A.D. – "That potion is snake oil, swallow this pill."
> 1985 A.D. – "That pill is ineffective, take this antibiotic."
> 2000 A.D. – "That antibiotic is artificial. Here, eat this root!"

What Types of Pain?

The accompanying brief descriptions might help us to quickly understand the nature of a patient's description:

1. **sharp** – quick, sticking, intense

2. **throbbing** – usually from an inflammation, adjacent

to an artery

3.   **dull** – not as intense or acute as *sharp*, possibly more annoying than painful

4.   **diffuse** – covering a large area

5.   **shifting** – moving from one area to another

6.   **intermittent** – coming and going

7.   **boring** – of an excruciating nature, usually in a bone

8.   **gnawing** – severe type of pain, usually that of a tumour invading surrounding tissue

9.   **aching** – over-action of a weak part or muscle

10. **spasm** – like a 'stitch', caused by violent exercise

11. **griping** – agonising pain, caused by irritation of bowels, bile-ducts, ureters, etc.

12. **burning** – certain types of dyspepsia, due to the action of excessive acid, gastric juice, and burns of skin

13. **referred pain** – experienced in part of body that is not the place of injury or disease, e.g. people with gallbladder disease often complain of pain in upper back or shoulder

14. **phantom pain** – pain felt in an amputated extremity (which proves that pain can be felt without having tissue damage and without nerve roots from the painful area to the brain)

15. **vascular pain** – very severe pain arising when the

blood supply to tissues, especially with muscles, is cut off

16. **headache pain** – because it is such a common symptom in so many diseases, it would be of little value to list all the causes here. There is a special section on this subject. Certain diseases, however, have headaches as a presenting symptom, and these include:

> all forms of meningitis and encephalitis
>
> cerebral tumours, abscesses and aneurysms
>
> diseases of the nasal and paranasal sinuses
>
> hypertension (in some cases headache might be slight)
>
> migraine.

These descriptions of pain are essential in helping a therapist to make an accurate diagnosis of the probable underlying cause, which could be any of the following:

Nociceptive – most common categories are *thermal* – caused by excessive heat or cold, *mechanical* – crushing, tearing, piercing (by pin, splinter, nail, knife, etc.) and *chemical* – iodine in a cut, pepper in the eyes, etc.

Inflammatory – usually characterised by hotness, swelling and redness and can include any of the following: autoimmune disease, pelvic inflammatory disease, rheumatoid arthritis, vasculitis, disc herniation or degeneration, ankylosing spondylitis, scoliosis or compression fracture, to name just a few.

Neuropathic – sensations of burning, tingling, stabbing, pins and needles, trapped nerves (e.g. sciatica) etc. Can be the result of post-shingles, neuralgia, nerve compression from tumour, injury, malfunction of Central Nervous System (CNS), strangulation by scar tissue, inflamed by infection, and can last for days, weeks, months or years.

Psychogenic – this is a back pain disorder brought about by psychological or emotional factors. It can cause, increase or even prolong pain. It can often be distinguished from other causes of pain because the symptoms might well not match the patient's complaint.

Adaptive, Protective – a person with back pain, especially lumbar pain, may adopt a change of posture which enables them to stand, sit or walk a little more comfortably. A typical example of upper back pain adaptation is the stoop.

How Does Pain Affect Us?

Pain doesn't affect everybody in the same way, for a variety of reasons. So let's ask how it affects YOU.

- Do you find the pain distracts from concentrating on what you should be doing?
- Does it make you feel grumpy and irritable?

- Does it make you feel bitter?

- Do you ever ask, 'Why me?'

- If you get pain spasms in public do you find it embarrassing that people might think you are drunk?

- Has pain made you turn to alcohol to get relief?

- Do you feel like crying or screaming out in frustration at your inability to find pain relief?

- Are you becoming more prone to fits of depression as your pain continues?

- Have you even felt suicidal?

- Do you sometimes lie in a darkened room to shut yourself off from the rest of the world?

- Do you fear that your spine is crumbling and you will become a cripple?

- Do you find it almost impossible to get a decent night's sleep?

- Do you get feelings of despair followed by an impulse to panic?

- Has your pain deeply affected your sex life?

- Do you fear losing your job or business because of your frequent loss of working days?

- Has your pain affected your ability to interact with

others?

- Have you started putting on weight as a direct result of your pain?

- Do you start getting anxious about the even the smallest things?

- Do you think colleagues and friends think you are 'putting it on'?

- Do you sometimes feel your doctor is failing to understand what you are going through?

- Have you come to believe that your pain is now permanent?

The list could go on and on. The reality is that back pain can be frightening, frustrating, debilitating and depressing. Above all, you want rid of it! And fast.

The next section deals with the mechanics of pain, which is designed to help you understand what causes the pain and why. I would advise you to read through it quickly, but if your pain is so intense you want to move through to the following section on treatment SOLUTIONS I would fully understand.

THE MECHANICS of PAIN

Why and How it Occurs

We used to think about what pain is, how the body perceives it, how we can treat it mechanically and chemically. At the risk of oversimplifying this, let me give you the conclusion first:

> 'If there was no pain there would be no doctors. The relief of pain was the prime objective of the doctor to improve his patient's quality of life. And since pain is experienced as an emotion, pain removal becomes an important mental goal in improving the quality of life.'

Patients probably go to doctors more commonly for pain relief than for any other reason. The average patient says, 'It hurts here, it hurts there. Give me something to stop the pain.' Pain is what primarily brings them to the office. Pain, discomfort, and dysfunction. The doctor is judged, oftentimes, by his success in relieving pain.

It's often considered that the best pain explanation we have is the Melzack Wall Gate Theory of Pain, which I touched on in the previous section.

These were two researchers who came up with the theory of a spinal gate concept of pain, and basically what they said is, there's a spinal gate that switches back and forth from the large neuro-fibres to the small neuro-fibres. And pain is produced when the gate switches to one direction and pain can be relieved when you can get the gate to switch back to the other direction. *And it doesn't matter which position it was in to start with.*

Part of the explanation is that when you bump your knee and it hurts like crazy, you can rub your knee and make the pain diminish – because the rubbing sensation goes to the brain on a different nerve fibre than the pain sensation – that diminishes the brain's sensation.

That has been the main pain explanation for many years. But even at best, it was just a theory.

Now, other researchers are saying that's a bunch of baloney. That's <u>not</u> the way the body perceives pain.

In the opening paragraph of this section, I gave you the *conclusion* of an article. The opening sentence of the article is, 'The Malzack Wall Theory of Pain is dead.' Long live the new neurology of pain.

So what is this new neurology? You understand that we have all kinds of nerve endings in our body and those nerve endings measure temperature, pressure and sensation. We have special sensations in our body that measure sound, hearing, taste, smell and vision. But you notice there are no organs specifically for pain only. There are no nerve endings for pain only.

You cannot pinpoint a certain place in the body and say 'this anatomical structure right here is for the purpose of registering pain.' We don't have pain nerve endings, or a special sense for pain only. We have sensory nerves that relay information back to the brain allowing us to experience pain, but these nerves are specifically *pain* nerves.

So the most revolutionary thing I'm going to tell you is that pain is perceived in the *emotional* part of the brain. In the frontal cortex of the limbic system.

What does all that mean in common language? It means **pain is an emotional experience**.

An emotional experience that can be brought about by several different methods. But if it is an emotional experience rather than a cut and dried physiological process (a switch flipping from one position to another position), it greatly changes our approach in the way we treat it, and how we perceive it.

You understand that you have to have a new concept about something *before* you can deal with it. And how you deal with it depends on your concept of it.

So, to summarise what I've said so far, it boils down to this: we experience pain, we are aware of pain, but technically we do not sense pain. And I don't want this to be a play on words only. We do not sense pain like we sense hearing or sight. We experience pain, we are aware of pain, and pain results in an activation of certain neurons in the brain – in the area of the cerebral cortex of the limbic system.

Let me jump ahead and give you an example. Don't we all know of experiences that we have either heard of or had ourselves? Where people have been subjected to some kind of trauma where they should have been in immense pain? Like the soldier on the battlefield who got his arm blown off and he kept walking – he didn't even know his arm was missing! How can we explain that? That's proof right there that the body is more powerful than just a pain being an automatic phenomenon.

Pain is experienced, we become aware of pain, but there are certain requirements for us to become aware of it. And if these requirements are not there then we're *not* aware of it. And because individuals vary, so does the pain *threshold* vary between individuals.

Pain is experienced through several methods.

One is a mechanical deformation of the sensory nerve endings from physical sources, such as trauma, pressure, a pin prick. In other words, these nerve endings can become physically deformed by some type of trauma that can alter the nerve ending which sends a message to the brain, and we become aware of pain as a result of that trauma.

Another way we experience pain is a chemical reaction. In other words, the nerve endings can become depolarised – which means activated by a chemical reaction. The reaction could be thermo-stimulation, but most often it is due to a chemical change.

To simplify it, there are basically only 6 chemicals that can cause this. And 4 of these chemicals are the result of inflammation in the body. *Inflammatory responses*. The other two are the result of muscular fatigue.

In other words, muscular fatigue can cause the production of chemicals that can lead to a depolarisation of the nociceptors.

These are the 6 chemicals that are in the body that are capable of depolarising the nociceptors (the nerves that *perceive* pain):

- Histamine
- Prostaglandins
- Kinins
- Serotonin
- Potassium ions
- Lactic acid

Three of these chemicals, histamine, kinins and prostaglandins are also neuro-transmitters.

What I'm saying is that if we can control these substances in the body we can control pain.

So the new functional neurology of pain is now

something that we can sink our teeth into, that we can do something with. With the Malzack Wall Theory we were helpless most of the time. There was no effective way of preventing the spinal gate flipping back and forth – although acupuncture did offer some relief.

Now we can do something about this.

If our goal is to control pain, we have to consider all aspects of the generation and transmission of the nerve impulses that result in pain. And that would include an evaluation of the body's chemistry to determine if there's a chemical basis for the pain.

Doesn't all this sound like an over-simplification of pain? Of course it does, and you're quite right if you thought it. I agree with elements of this new concept, but it doesn't take into account other things that we know about pain.

I'm going to discuss a whole lot of different issues throughout this book, but we have to start somewhere, don't we? Let's take a different view now.

Pain appears to have 3 components:

1. a stimulus, physical or mental

2. a physical sensation of hurting

3. the reaction of the person experiencing it.

Before we can offer any kind of treatment we have to

make a number of assessments based on what a person tells us, any behaviour responses we can observe, and some knowledge of the physiological, psychological, cultural, environmental and nutritional aspects of the individual patient.

We can learn most of that from asking the right questions, and I have prepared a questionnaire that I developed for patients at my Pain Clinic in London.

Let's take a look at the functions of pain.

1.   as an adaptation for protection against injury

2.   to inform us that something is amiss

3.   as an indirect aid in the repair and replacement of damaged tissue.

With regard to #1, because of pain we may decide to move away from the painful stimuli, or we may learn to prevent a recurrence of the injury.

In #2, slight pain warns us of slight damage, which may then be attended to before more serious damage results – i.e. pain tells us that a tooth is decaying, and we attend to it before an abscess forms. Pain not only warns us of trouble but often tells us where the trouble is, i.e. tells you which finger has a splinter in it. It is also one of the most important symptoms of disease, and we can learn a great deal from knowing exactly what type of pain is present and where it is located.

In #3, rest is often the best single aid to healing. Pain often enforces rest; if severe enough, it may impose absolute rest in bed, or merely enforce rest of the injured part, i.e. it immobilises a broken arm, facilitating the growth of new bone, which heals the fracture. Current medical thinking is that bed rest is inadvisable in cases of back pain and can actually make it worse.

Pain has various characteristics, e.g. there may or may not be damage to body tissue when pain occurs. The pain of grief can cause mental suffering that does not involve tissue damage. The amount of pain is not necessarily in proportion to the amount of damage occurring in the body.

Some people experience the pain of anticipation, e.g. the misery of anticipating pain when the dentist is about to drill and repair a cavity. People also view pain differently, e.g. some may wish to be thought of as brave and sturdy, and may therefore describe their pain casually as though it hardly existed, even when it is considerable; another person may show great concern and anxiety when the pain is minor. In other words, we can't always make an accurate assessment based on a patient's own description.

A patient may experience any one or all of the following phases of a pain experience:

1.   the anticipation of pain

2. the sensation of pain

3. the aftermath of pain

In helping a person cope with pain we need to recognise which of the above 3 phases he/she is in. Ideally, we can help most when he/she is in the first phase, since we can begin to condition him/her favourably for the other two phases.

When a person has pain, he/she usually exhibits non-verbal signs, which we should be able to recognise; a person may frown, grimace or cry; he/she may pace the floor, grip onto a bed or chair, or clench jaws or fist; he/she may show signs of anger, fear, frustration or worry; or there may be tense, firm muscles in the affected area.

There are also signs that the patient cannot control; pulse and respiratory rates will increase, blood pressure may be elevated, or he/she may faint; the pupils might become dilated.

Many experiments have been conducted on animals to test whether endorphins and enkephalins (pain-killing hormones produced in the brain) can be artificially stimulated and released. While this has been successfully done on rats, mice and cats, it must be remembered that when applying the same concept to humans we have to take into account the complex psychological factors that surround pain.

It is useful to think of pain perception as a complex interaction between the physical stimulus that causes the pain and the psychological reactive component to it, sometimes called the 'hurt'.

In most clinical pain situations, the physical component fortunately is not so severe that it saturates the entire perceptual channel, leaving no room for the reactive component, the hurt. When the physical stimulus causing pain is that intense, it often leads to surgical shock, or other kinds of unconsciousness. Should the patient retain consciousness with an overwhelming physical pain – e.g. passing a renal stone, suffering acute pancreatitis, or receiving a crushing blow to a limb – psychological factors are of minimal importance in controlling the pain. However, in most clinical pain situations, the reactive component *is* important and provides greater flexibility in the perception of the pain.

A classic example is to compare soldiers wounded in battle with a matched group of surgical patients in a general hospital. Beecher (1966) found that the soldiers reported minimal pain and rarely requested pain medication – even when faced with appalling physical injuries – whereas the surgical patients demanded drugs for pain relief.

The soldiers were grateful to be alive and wished to remain as sharp and alert as possible in order to continue being alive. They also saw it as a way out of the war, since they would expect to be repatriated home. Consequently, they processed their pain stimulus very differently from the surgical patients, to whom pain represented an interference in the flow of their lives.

What causes back pain?

There is an overlap between the network of small and large nerves that cover the entire body, none more so than those surrounding the vertebrae (backbone). This can make it difficult for a sufferer to describe his/her precise location of pain. However, the main causes of spinal injuries are:

- The bones, joints and ligaments (a band of fibrous tissue connecting bones or cartilages, serving to support and strengthen joints) may be damaged or compressed.

- A herniated or ruptured disc (often called a 'slipped disc'), commonly caused when bending awkwardly, lifting, twisting or by direct injury to the spine – as in a fall or some kind of accident. Other causes can be long-term smoking, overweight, jobs that involve a lot of sitting. What happens is that after rupturing, some of the gelatinous content of the disc squeezes out (like toothpaste from a tube) and presses on a spinal nerve, causing acute pain.

- Strain to the back muscles (shown in diagram below). Muscle strain pain tends to clear up reasonably quickly.

- Irritation to large nerve roots that go to arms and legs, usually due to some kind of inflammation.

- Some of the smaller nerve roots of the spine can be irritated, also usually as the result of inflammation.

- Spinal stenosis, often due to arthritis causing a constriction of muscles supporting the spine.

- Osteoporosis, a weakening of the bones, can lead to fractures of the spine.

- Poor posture – sitting, standing, sleeping or walking – often causes backache and pain.

CERVICAL BACK PAIN SOLUTIONS –

Made Simple

You are about to receive a cascade of solutions to the various kinds of cervical back pain problems. Some – many, in fact – you will be able to do on your own. A few may require the assistance of someone else. Even fewer might require professional attention.

Solutions, or treatments, cannot start until we know exactly where the pain is, and what type of pain it is. For our purpose, I am going to subdivide back pain into three sections:

1. Cervical – neck

2. Thoracic – main trunk of the spine

3. Lumbar – lower end of the spine, including the coccyx (tailbone)

It is estimated that about 75% of all adults will experience low back pain at some time during their life. The most common age span for this condition is 30-40 years of age.

Statistically, 60% of people will first see their general practitioner, 25% will see a specialist in back pain, and 15% will see an osteopath or chiropractor. Lifting injuries accounts for 49%, twisting for 18%, and bending is associated with 12%. Reaching, arching, pulling or pushing accounts for the remainder.

In the UK, about 18 million working-days are lost per year, making it the number one cause of lost working days. If the patient has suffered with the problem for 3 months or less it is regarded as *acute*, and for more than 3 months is said to be *chronic*. About 75% of all acute problems usually heal and return to normal within two months. Chronic pain can last for months or even years and is the most difficult to treat. Difficult, but not impossible, as we shall see.

Pain Tracing

Because pain sensations sometimes come and go (intermittent) or may be some distance away from the actual location of the injury or disease (referred), it is useful to locate the real source (pain epicentre). A medical doctor will usually determine the source of the pain by having x-rays, CT (Computerized tomography) or MRI (Magnetic Resonance Imaging) scans carried out. An EMG (Electromyography) test can show if compressions of the nerves are present, or a bone scan can reveal tumours or spinal compressions. The self-helper, or the *alternative practitioner*, doesn't have that luxury – if subjecting the body to unnatural bombardment of harmful rays can be called a luxury. *But that's another subject!*

When we need to know if the pain is referred from another source or if the pain just feels as if it's moving around, we can use a technique I call Pain Tracing. We can do this by getting a patient to deeply relax. I know! It's difficult to relax when you're suffering a great deal of pain, but you can try as much as possible. Best done if patients sits or lies comfortably with eyes closed, and taking a few deep breaths. Then ask patient to put an index finger firmly on the point where pain is felt – without applying pressure – and counting up to 10. If pain has moved, then patient again places finger of other hand on new pain point before moving first finger, and again counts up to 10. Repeat this as often as necessary until the pain ceases to move to another place. This final place is the *epicentre,* from which the pain is emanating.

Below is a facsimile of the actual sheet I gave to patients attending my Pain Clinic in London.

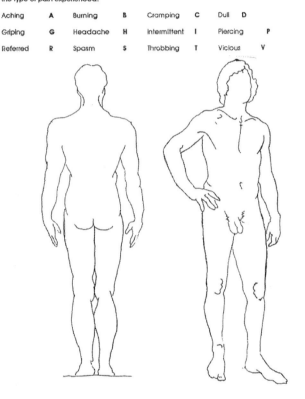

In order to help us quickly diagnose your painful condition, please mark the diagrams below to indicate where you have had pain, now or in the past, using the following symbols to indicate the type of pain experienced:

Aching	A	Burning	B	Cramping	C	Dull	D
Griping	G	Headache	H	Intermittent	I	Piercing	P
Referred	R	Spasm	S	Throbbing	T	Vicious	V

Use this pain scale to indicate the severity of your pain.

If a zero (0) means 'no pain' and a ten (10) means 'pain as bad as it can be', on this scale of 0 to 10 what is your level of pain?

| 0 | 1 | 2 | 3 | 4 | 5 | 6 | 7 | 8 | 9 | 10 |

And because it wouldn't be nice to ask a female to fill in her pain points on a male figure, I also gave out a different chart to female patients, as shown below:

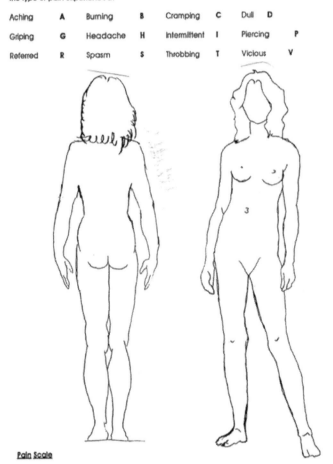

Instructions for Patient

Where is the pain? What is the pain like? How severe is the pain?

In order to help us quickly diagnose your painful condition, please mark the diagrams below to indicate where you have had pain, now or in the past, using the following symbols to indicate the type of pain experienced:

Aching	A	Burning	B	Cramping	C	Dull	D
Griping	G	Headache	H	Intermittent	I	Piercing	P
Referred	R	Spasm	S	Throbbing	T	Vicious	V

Pain Scale

Pain Questionnaire

Before we can begin looking for the right solution we need more information about the pain. I used to give the following questionnaire out to patients while they were in the waiting room so that no time would be lost during our session together.

TYPES OF PAIN

It is useful to know the different types of pain, and the accompanying brief list with descriptions may help us to quickly identify and understand the nature of your condition:

Sharp – quick, sticking, intense

Throbbing – usually from an inflammation

Dull – not as intense or acute as sharp, possibly more annoying than painful

Diffuse – covering a large area

Shifting – moving from area to another

Intermittent – coming and going

Boring – of an excruciating character, usually in bone

Gnawing – severe type of pain, usually that of a tumour invading surrounding tissue

Aching – over-action of a weak part or muscle

Spasm – like a 'stitch', usually caused by violent exercise

Griping – agonising pain, caused by irritation of bowel, bile duct, etc.

Burning – certain types of dyspepsia, due to the action of excessive acid, gastric juice, and burns of skin

Referred pain – pain experienced in a part of the body which is not the place of injury or disease, e.g. people with gallbladder disease often complain of pain in upper back or shoulder

Phantom pain – pain in an amputated extremity (which proves that pain can be felt without having damaged tissue and without nerve roots from the painful area to the brain. This indicates that the sufferer is experiencing 'mental' pain

Vascular pain very severe pain arising when the blood supply to tissues, especially muscles, is cut off

GENERAL QUESTIONS

1. Do you get any pain in joints or muscles? If so, which?

2. How much alcohol do you drink daily? Weekly?

3. Do you smoke? If yes, how many per day? Week?

4. Do you exercise regularly? What kind of exercise, typically?

5. Are you under any excessive stress?

6. Is your work mainly sedentary?

7. Does your work involve much lifting of heavy goods?

8. Do you work with heavy machinery?

9. Over what period have you had your pain? Is it constant, or does it come and go?

Okay. You should by now know precisely where the pain is located, and the nature of the pain. That is, whether it is anatomic – the result of a physical injury or damage – chemical – caused by something eaten, swallowed, applied to the skin (some kind of balm or cream, or even soap – or if it is psychological/emotional – caused by the memory of something painful that is still causing distress and pain.

The Muscle Test

We will use the names *testee* for person being tested, and *testor* for the partner doing the testing. So, standing facing each other, testee raises arm level with shoulder (either arm can be used). Testor places one hand just above the testee's wrist and the other hand on the opposing shoulder just to make contact. Think of it as being an electrical circuit – which is what it is – in which you have a positive and a negative wire; if only one wire makes contact with the electrical source no energy is passed – contact must be made with both wires in order for electrical energy to flow. The body is similar.

So, placing the hand lightly on the shoulder – being careful not to exert pressure – and the other hand above the testee's wrist, a little pressure is gently exerted to push the outstretched arm in a downward direction. **Important note:** this is not a test of strength. The object is not to try and force the testee's arm down, merely to see if there is a little *give* in the arm. Without a challenge – which we'll come to in a moment – the testee's arm should remain level with the shoulder as a gentle pressure is applied. This is normal.

The **challenge** comes in some form from the testor. For example, if something *toxic* – like a small battery – is placed in the hand of the testee, and the outstretched arm is then pressed lightly down (about 4 lb pressure is enough in most cases), the outstretched arm will almost certainly be much weaker and might even completely collapse. This is because the energy field of the battery has negatively affected the muscle being tested – the *deltoid* in this case – causing the muscle mass to lose its strength.

Remove the battery from the other hand and test the muscle again and it should have regained its full strength, so the weakness is only momentary.

The opposite can occur in some cases. For example, when the outstretched arm goes weak when tested, placing a sachet of sugar in the other hand and then retesting the muscle might cause it to regain its strength. This is because the energy from the sugar might be *positively* enhancing the strength of the deltoid muscle. If sugar doesn't strengthen the muscle, various substances can be placed in the hand – one at a time, of course – until something is found that enhances the strength. Remember this: nothing works for everybody! So we can generalise and say do this or do that, but in rare cases we might find the opposite effect is happening. This is where the experience of the testor is invaluable. But it doesn't alter the fact that in most cases, the procedure will follow that outlined above. A little practice will give confidence and assurance to testee and testor in the early stages.

Getting to understand this simple test and conduct it with ease will be so valuable, as we will progressively see, because you will be able to apply it to a rich variety of instances where this simple muscle test will reveal why things have been working or <u>not</u> working for you in the past. It is like having a magic entry into the strange workings of the body and mind.

So now we can do the basic muscle test and we are ready to apply it to your back pain. And we are going to do it in a slightly different way. The testee – the person with the pain – is going to lie down in a supine (on his/her back) position. Raising the arm level with the shoulder but forward of the body rather than sideways to it. The testor will stand to the side and place a hand above the wrist – exactly as when down in a standing position – but the other hand will be placed lightly on the mid thigh rather than on the opposing shoulder. This is purely for the sake of convenience. And to test the muscle, a little pressure will be applied to push the outstretched arm down towards the feet. The muscle should be strong at this stage.

Next, the testee will place a finger on the part of the back where the pain is felt. The testor then pushes down on the arm. If the muscle goes weak, this indicates that there is physical damage to that part of the being tested. If the muscle remains strong, we now do something different. The testee puts his/her head in extension – meaning that the neck is stretched back so that the head is resting on its crown.

Then the muscle is tested again. If the muscle now goes weak this is an indication that the pain is of a psychological or emotional nature. And the treatment is extremely simple and extremely effective.

Let the head return to its normal resting position. Throughout this whole procedure, the testee must have his/her finger remaining in position on the location on that part of spine giving pain. Before the treatment is started, it is **very** helpful to get a good indicator of the level of pain the testee is feeling. I use what I call the Personal Assessment Scale (PAS), asking the patient to express their assessment on a scale of 1-10, with 1 meaning very little pain and 10 indicating the worst possible pain.

Let's say, in our example, the patient says 8, meaning very acute pain.

Treatment Mode

1. Testor stands at the head of the table couch where the testee is lying.

2. Very gently – and it should be stressed to the testee that this **is** a very gentle procedure which will not give any pain or discomfort, and it is important for the testee to just relax the muscles and allow the testor to proceed – the testor cradles both hands together and gently slides them under the testee's head.

3. The testor now very gently flexes the testee's head – that is, lifts it so that it is pointing towards the feet. No force should be used and the range of movement will probably be no more than a few inches.

4. Just as gently, the testor lowers the head back to its resting position.

5. After about three deep breaths, the procedure two more times in exactly the same way.

6. After a brief relaxation period – maybe 15-20 seconds – the head is tested again by going into extension as before. The muscle is tested again. If the muscle, which previously went weak when the head was in extension, is now testing strong, this is an indication that the treatment has been completed successfully.

The patient can now remove his/her finger from the point of pain location and place their arm down by their side. He/she is now asked how the pain would be expressed on the PAS. Much depends on the answer. It may be for example 4. Now to go from an 8 to a 4 is a considerable improvement, but it wouldn't satisfy me. I would want to get it down to a very minimum of 1, or even 0. If it had gone from an 8 to a 7 or 6, then I would consider that nothing has been achieved.

From experience I can say that in the vast majority of cases I have done, using this technique – which I call *Trauma Delete* – the pain has completely gone. In a minority of cases I have had to repeat the treatment procedure maybe two more times. Remember that the testee has to place his/her finger on the point where pain is felt. In some cases, I have found that the pain is no longer in the original place and the testee has to find another spot where pain is detected. Then the whole procedure of testing and treatment is repeated. At the end of each treatment session, remember to check the PAS because there is no other way of making an assessment of any residual pain.

Trauma Delete is the most successful way of eliminating pain that I know of. I have used it on **thousands** of people around the world and have never had a single failure anywhere. I haven't, in every case, been able to completely remove all pain but I have in every case been able to reduce it to at least an acceptable level. It has always been time that has prevented me from removing it completely.

Before my retirement, I gave a demonstration in Sri Lanka in front of 5,000 people, allowing *anyone* in the audience to come and be tested/treated. It lasted for several hours and was videotaped throughout. I had one girl who had fallen and broken her ankle that very morning. Within 10 minutes all pain was completely removed and the swelling reduced remarkably.

In Lisbon, at the end of a World Conference on Medical Science, I was approached by a guy – he was Scandinavian – who told me he had been an Olympic athlete whose career had been curtailed by an injury to his leg. He had explored every medical avenue with no success and no prospect for success. Could I help? I looked around and everyone was departing the venue – the Penta Hotel Conference Hall. I said I would like to but there wasn't even a table for him to lie on. He said he would lie on the floor. Not wanting to disappoint him, I agreed. So kneeling on the floor beside him, I carried out the procedure outlined above. At the end of it he jumped up in joy, thrusting his body and legs in various positions trying to see if he could bring the pain back. Which he couldn't. He threw his arms round me and said, 'You have resurrected my Olympic career!' I never saw him again. I don't even know his name. So whether he actually made it to the next Olympics I will probably never know. I hope he did.

Okay, so now we are ready to start looking at solutions for the three designated areas I mentioned earlier, cervical, thoracic or lumbar regions of the back.

Cervical Pain

The cervical area of the spine is represented by the diagram below, shown in red, and its function is to support the head and to contain and support the spinal cord. It consists of seven vertebrae identified as C1, C2, C3, C4, C5, C6, and C7. This unique structure allows the head to tilt backwards (extension, already mentioned) or forwards (flexion), or sideways (rotation).

The cervical spine is supported and stabilised by a complex system of ligaments – a band of tough fibrous fibres which join one bone to another bone – tendons – a band of inelastic fibres which connect a muscle to a bone – and muscles, which can contract and relax under the direction of nerve impulses relayed from the brain. As well as providing support and stability, it is muscles which allow mobility. Most muscles in the body work as pairs, meaning that as one muscle contracts the opposing muscle relaxes.

Nerve impulses are carried along the spinal cord by a system called the *Peripheral Nervous System* (PNS). These nerves spread from their spinal root throughout the body in the following direction:

C1 and C2 – to the head and neck

C3 – to the diaphragm

C4 – upper body muscles i.e. deltoids – which I commonly use for muscle testing

C5 and C6 – wrist extensors

C7 – triceps (that run along the back of the upper arm and allow the raising and lowering of the forearm)

Most of the rotation is facilitated at C1(called the *atlas*) and C2 (called the *axis*) level, while extension and flexion takes place through C5-C6, and C6-C7. The body had what is called *righting reflexes* so that if we lean too much to either side opposing muscles prevent us from falling over.

Each spinal segment includes two vertebrae separated by an intervertebral disc, which acts as a kind of shock absorber.

The facet joints are joined together rather like a chain, and the total is called the spinal column, or backbone or spine. The inside of the intervertebral disc contains a mucoprotein gel. If the disc should be damaged or herniated, this gel is likely to squeeze out (like toothpaste from a tube), where it can compress against a nerve causing excruciating pain.

Pain can also be caused by what is commonly known as a *degeneration* of the vertebrae, although that has not been satisfactorily defined. It is generally thought to be brought about by normal wear and tear, although damage or injury to the spine can bring it about. The main symptom is a *stiff neck* or loss of range of motion. When trying to determine the cause, a good indicator is how it affects other parts of the body. Using the guide given above, we can say that if the stiff neck is also affecting the movement of either or both wrists then C5-C6 is likely to be involved. Or if it affects the ability to raise the forearm easily, then C6-C7 could be involved. A simple muscle test to either of these points could be used to confirm this.

X-rays or an MRI or CT scan might reveal calcification of one or more joints, or even the early stages of arthritis.

Another cause of head and neck pain can be cancer, which can be in several different forms:

Burkitt's lymphoma, in which white blood cells – called *lymphocytes* – behave abnormally and form together in clumps. Medical treatment should be sought for this, although alternative treatments might well complement that.

Hodgkin's disease, affects lymph nodes in the head or neck and is caused by abnormalities of lymphocytes. This can spread quickly from one lymph to another. Again, medical attention should be sought for any kind of cancer, although alternative treatments are sometimes available which might complement any medical treatment – which would probably be radiotherapy or chemotherapy.

Whiplash, most commonly caused through motor accidents, is another debilitating neck injury that can cause acute pain and restriction of movement of the head and neck.

Spinal stenosis is a narrowing of the spinal canal, which carries the nerves. As well as pain, a common symptom is numbness or *paraesthesia*. This can affect the whole body, even causing paralysis in extreme cases.

SOLUTIONS

Before giving solutions there are a couple of points important to understand and remember:

1. Pain is a messenger, not an injury or disease in itself. It merely informs us that something is wrong, either damage or out of balance in some way.

2. Removing the pain, which is what the solutions are aimed at, does not repair the injury or imbalance.

3. If you have any doubts about any of the solutions suggested below, seek advice from an appropriate professional, i.e. kinesiologist, osteopath, chiropractor, nutritionist, homeopath, herbalist, physiotherapist, or GP.

Whiplash

Most commonly caused by a car accident or by any jolt to the head from behind.

The term whiplash is not, in itself, a diagnosis, nor is it an accurate description of the type of injury incurred. It would be more accurate to describe it as either a hyperextension or a hyperflexion of the head and neck, meaning that the head and neck have been forced backwards or forwards beyond their natural range of mobility.

TRAUMA DELETE

This is the treatment of choice, from *Myoneurology*, and in the vast majority of cases will remove the pain within minutes – if carried out correctly. Remember to ask degree of pain experienced on the PAS level of 1-10 before commencing treatment.

1. Locate the point of injury – most commonly between C5-C6. Testee places finger on that point.

2. Test muscle. Should be strong.

3. Put head into extension.

4. Test muscle. If weak, means you have the right spot for treatment. If strong, move finger to a slightly different location and repeat test.

5. Once you have found the location which causes a weak muscle, with testee's finger remaining on same spot, testor places both hands beneath head and neck and gently puts the head forward into flexion – lifting as far forward as possible without causing additional pain or discomfort. Repeat this flexion 5 times.

6. Testee removes hands and tests muscle again with head in extension. Should now be strong. If still weak, put head and neck into flexion another 3 times and retest.

If the muscle now tests strong, ask patient to assess pain level on the PAS scale. If treatment is successful, there should be a considerable – if not complete – reduction of pain. If not completely removed, do the whole test and treatment again, only with testee moving finger to another point – probably C6-C7.

Once that treatment has been successfully completed, it is advisable to give back-up support in the nature of nutrition – to help repair any damaged tissue caused by the whiplash injury – or herbs, homeopathy, VibroFusion, etc.

NUTRITION

The nutritional support suggested below might seem daunting if you feel that you should need all of them. Not the case. Common sense needs to be applied, e.g. if there is little or no swelling at the site of injury, it shouldn't be necessary to take something to reduce swelling. If unsure, contact a local nutritionist for advice. Health food shops, Yellow Pages, etc. can help you find one if you are unsure. Personal recommendations are always the best, of course.

Proteolytic enzymes help digest proteins, necessary for repair of damaged tissue. They also help reduce pain and swelling from joint inflammation. Holland & Barrett have a selection of low-priced enzymes. Amazon also offers a wide range of enzymes.

Vitamins A and D support healing of bone fractures

Vitamin B complex helps repair injured muscles and connective tissue

Vitamin B$_1$ helps reduce chronic nerve and bone pain and also helps alleviate headaches arising from whiplash injury

Magnesium helps relax stiff and taut muscles

Calcium is good for nerve conduction and bone health, as well as helping reduce pain arising from any swelling

Zinc supports protein synthesis necessary for tissue repair, and also helps strengthen the immune system

Manganese provides good healing support for damage to tendons and ligaments

Glucosamine and Chondroitin help rebuild damaged cartilage, where this has occurred

Foods that might help include nuts, oats, muesli, sunflower seeds and green leafy vegetables.

HERBS

Can often be purchased either loose or in capsule form from health food shops. National suppliers are G. Baldwin & Co., The Organic Herb Trading Co., R & G Fresh Herbs, Abbey Botanicals Herbs & Spices, White Tiger Medicine, amongst many herbal suppliers throughout the world. Or contact a local medical herbalist for advice.

Gotu Kola *(Centella asiatica)* helps heal connective tissue, i.e. tendons, ligaments, by stimulating collagen synthetis

Kava Kava *(Piper methysticum)* helps reduce nerve pain and inflammation. Also helps with headaches

Arnica *(Arnica Montana)* helps reduce swelling, pain and inflammation due to injury

Devil's Claw *(Harpagophytum procumbens)* helps reduce inflammation and pain, especially nerve pain. Claimed by some herbalists to be superior to cortisone

Frankincense *(Boswellia serrate)* reduces swelling pain and stiffness. Also improves blood circulation necessary to support tissue repair

Turmeric *(Curcuma longa)* anti-inflammatory, reduces swelling and pain

St John's Wort *(Hypericum perforatum)* good for nerve pain, swelling and muscle aches

HOMEOPATHY

Symphytum Officinale facilitates of fractured or damaged bone, joints and cartilage

Ruta Graveolens helps repair injuries, especially of joints and tendons

Arnica Montana is one of homeopathy's great healers, especially good for injuries to all soft tissue resulting from whiplash. Helps recovery from traumatic shock, concussion

Hypericum Perforatum often known as 'the arnica of the nerves' because of its ability to heal injured areas involving nerves and sensitive tissue. Particularly good for whiplash injury, concussion, and damage to the cervical spine

Suppliers in the UK include Nelsons UK, Ainsworths, and Enzyme Process, amongst many others. It is worth noting that a wide range of pharmacies throughout the country have been licensed by the Department of Health to supply homeopathic remedies. Always best to consult a homeopath before buying these inexpensive remedies.

VIBROFUSION (VF)

See Appendix A for information about suppliers and also about the products themselves.

H224 Pain #1 helps relieve cervical pain due to whiplash injury

H896 Pathex helps eliminate pain and pathological conditions in cervical vertebrae

H6 Inflammex for relief of temporary swelling and inflammatory conditions

TRIGGER POINTS

Whiplash injury is caused by an over-stretching of muscles in the neck and shoulder regions. The three most common muscles involved are the *sternocleidomastoid, scalenes* and *trapezius.*

What is a trigger point? Basically, they are made up of taut nodules sometimes found in a muscle that should be easily palpable. Meaning you should be able to feel it if you allow your fingers to pass gently over the muscle until finding a kind of knot.

How to treat. Once a trigger point has been located, place a thumb against it and press – not too deeply as to cause pain but enough to be felt – for about 10 seconds. This can be done by oneself or by a friend or colleague. During those 10 seconds, try to relax and breathe deeply. Now try pressing a little deeper and repeat the process – for about 10 seconds, again.

That's all there is to it. After effective treatment, the

nodule should have diminished or even vanished. And any pain associated with that point should have evaporated.

ACUPUNCTURE/ACUPRESSURE

The following acupuncture points can be used for pain and stiffness in the neck and shoulders, torticollis (wry neck), cervical sprain and strain, rheumatoid arthritis of cervical spine and for cervical spondylosis:

Du 20	Baihui	Lu 7	Lieque
GB 20	Fengchi	GB 39	Xuanzhong
Du 14	Dazhui	UB 11	Dashui

In cases of very painful and acute stiff neck with difficulty of lateral rotation and flexion, strong manual stimulation should be given at:

SI 6	Yanglao	SI 3	Houxi (very painful)

Obviously, acupuncture is a highly skilled profession which should only be carried out by a suitably qualified acupuncturist. The use of needles usually gets the best results, but it is not the only way of using the centuries-old discovery of energy channels running through the body, access through specific points known as acupoints.

Acupressure is one such method, which can be

done by almost anyone without the use of needles. Some people use a blunt scapula-like instrument and press the rounded end of the instrument against the specific acupoint, holding it there for up to a minute. How much pressure is applied varies but should never incur any pain in the procedure.

Acutapping is another method, usually preferred by kinesologists and myoneurologists. Instead of using a blunt instrument the practitioner taps the acupoint in quick procession. I usually tap about 50 times. If this helps but doesn't completely remove the pain I might tap a further 50 or so times.

Remember the golden rule: nothing works for everyone. [Although as previously stated, I have never had a failure with *Trauma Delete*.] So the more tools you have available, the better the chance of success. Sometimes a combination of different treatment modes is necessary.

PSYCHOFUSION (PF)

This is a method I developed over many years, arising from my studies and research in clinical psychology and energy medicine. When dealing with some aspects of physical injury or damage it involves another personal development, *Quantum Vibes* (QV), which enables us to focus intense energy in quick, powerful bursts. The principles involve:

- Resonance

- Intention

- Attention (intense focus)

- Breathing in energy

- Innate body intelligence

It is something that can be done by the patient providing he/she is able to comfortably reach the place of injury with one hand. Place the thumb on one side of the injury and index and middle fingers together on the other side of the injury. Thus the injury is in between the thumb and other two fingers. Of course, if you cannot reach the point then you will need to recruit the help of someone else.

Once you have done this and can sit or lie in relative comfort close the eyes. I suggest this because it cuts out other stimuli which might interfere with your ability to concentrate fully on the task in hand. Once you are feeling relaxed – or the best you can do – breathe in deeply four or five times to establish a breathing rhythm. Then do the following:

1. Index and middle fingers on one side of the injury, thumb on the other side

2. Press more deeply as you breathe in

3. Simultaneously, focus your intention to heal

while you are breathing in

4. Relax fingers when breathing out

5. Maintain focus of intention and attention throughout

6. Press fingers more deeply as you start the next breathing cycle

7. Relax on breathing out

8. Repeat this cycle 5 times

9. Remove fingers and let the whole body relax

MAGNET THERAPY

This is something you can do yourself with very little effort. Of course, you will need magnets, and these are easily obtained for as little as £2.41 for a set of four. But first you need to know a couple of things about magnets in order to make the right purchase.

The type of magnet used for this purpose is made from an earth metal: *neodymion*. Magnets come in different sizes, shapes and strengths. Perhaps the best type for helping with neck pain are small, coin-shaped magnets with adhesive strips that enable them to be held firmly to the skin once placed in position. In common with other magnets, they have a North and South Pole, which is normally marked on the magnet.

*It is essential to use these Poles correctly as one can be healing and the other **harmful**.* More about this below. The strength of a magnet is measured in gauss and medical magnets can range in strength from 450 gauss to 10,000 gauss. As a general rule, the higher the gauss the better the pain relief.

It isn't necessary for you to know how and why magnets might relieve your pain. You probably want to get on with the treatment and get that relief. If so, go straight to the treatment section below. Others, however, prefer to know how something works in order to give credibility to the treatment. So for those, I will run through a potted version how the different parts of the body can be affected by magnetic polarity – remembering always that the North and South poles have different effects so great care needs to be taken when using magnets. *If in doubt, consult an expert.*

All cells in the body share common components, regardless of their type. One of the common constituents of all cells are ions. Ions are positively and negatively charged particles that conduct electro-magnetic pulses from within the cell. The electro-magnetic pulses allow the cell to function. Without ions, a cell cannot live.

In a normal healthy cell, the ions are distributed around the cell with all of the positive ions on one side and the negative ions on the opposing side. The ions which live outside of the cell in the tissues will align with those inside of the cell so that opposing poles are together with the cell membrane between them. This allows fluid, oxygen and nutrients (fluid exchange) to move freely in and out of the cell, while maintaining the natural balance within the cell (homeostasis).

In a diseased (injured) cell, the positive and negative ions do not stay on opposing sides of the cell. They are disrupted and scatter randomly around the cell. At the same time the ions on the outside of the cell membrane also become scattered as they try to find their opposing pole, this results in cellular imbalance. Extra fluid from the tissues outside the cell is able to penetrate the cell which in turn pushes vital nutrients, hormones and electrolytes (salts) out of the cell. The cell's ability to function is greatly reduced and cellular degeneration begins, which if not corrected will lead to the cell dying.

Conventional pain killing drugs like paracetamol and codeine based tablets (di-hydrocodiene, co codamol, co dydramol, tramadol and codeine phosphate) work by blocking the pain stimulus pathway. They interrupt the signal that starts at the point of pain (stimulus) and travel along the nerve pathways via the spinal cord to the pain receptors in the brain.

Depending on the type of drug, the signal may be interrupted at the pain stimulus or at any point along the nerve pathway to the brain. Pain killers only last for a short period of time. Depending on the type of pain killer and where they interrupt the pain pathway and the strength of the drug, they can last from 4-12 hours.

Magnets do not block the pain signal. They work on the cause of the pain, which is why static magnets have to be placed as close to the point of pain as possible.

Trauma alone does not cause all of the pain. Pain is also caused by pressure on the nerves. This can occur without a traumatic injury, as with long standing chronic conditions. Joint wear and tear, chronic damage from earlier injuries or chronic inflammation can cause pressure upon nerves. The pressure upon the nerves is usually caused by swelling or inflammation around the injury, this extra fluid causes the tissues to swell and thus places pressure upon the nerve endings. Compression of the nerves causes constant pain stimuli to be sent to the brain. This causes the chronic constant pain that is often associated with long term ailments.

To relieve the pressure on the compressed nerves the excess fluid in the tissues must be removed. Once the pressure has been removed the pain will subside. Magnets do reduce the inflammation in the tissues therefore they are very effective at reducing pain at the point of injury. Because the cause of the pain has been removed (i.e. the inflammation) the pain relieving results will last for a much longer period of time than pain killers, which are just blocking the signal. Whilst the magnetic field is reducing the inflammation it is also improving blood supply to the injured area. The extra blood flow brings fresh rich oxygen, nutrients and hormones. One of these hormones is endorphin. Endorphin is known as the "happy" hormone as it is responsible for mood enhancement. The other function of endorphin is to kill pain naturally. As increased blood flow reaches the injured area the concentration of endorphins increases and pain is reduced.

When the magnets are removed from the area of pain, the cause of the inflammation will return, as the magnets are a treatment for the inflammation and poor circulation, they are not a cure for any disease process. Depending on the severity of the injury or ailment the effects of the magnets can last days, weeks or even months. Each individual will experience different time scales for the return of the pain as the disease process for each individual is slightly different.

Magnetic fields will influence individual areas of the body in different ways. For example a swollen knee joint may respond very quickly to the presence of a magnetic field, with symptoms being alleviated with in just a few days. However the same person may treat another area of the body without the same quick response. The length of time that magnets will take to resolve the symptoms of an injury is entirely dependent on the severity of the ailment, the amount of inflammation surrounding the injured area, the cause of the ailment, and the type of magnets used. *Long standing chronic conditions, with large amounts of inflammation and cell damage will take longer to treat than a recent acute injury.*

The process is similar when looking at different people's reactions to magnets. Each individual will react to magnets in a slightly different way. Some people react very quickly to magnetic fields and others will take a longer period of time. An individual's medical history and symptoms must be taken into consideration when estimating how long magnets will take to work for a particular ailment.

Results can take anywhere from 2 days – 6 weeks depending on the condition and the severity of the injury.

North and South Poles have different effects

Magnetic Therapy in its natural state is the dominant North Pole field of the Earth dominating over the life processes of the body. With a full magnetic field from the

Earth the body goes through many actions to promote good growth, strengthen tissue and fight disease and damage from accidents or injury. However most of the Earth does not have a full magnetic field. Scientists tell us that as a normal process the Earth's poles reverse approximately every 5,000 years. This could explain the loss of a lot of dinosaur. As we move to this polarity switch, in about 2,000 years, the Earth's magnetic field is lessening. With a decreased field the body is not always able to make all the changes it should and it makes it unable to successfully protect itself. An interesting note is that there are only four places left on Earth with full magnetic fields. Two habitable and two are not. The *not* are the North Pole and the South Pole. The habitable are Sedona, Arizona and Lourdes, France – both known for healthy living and healing. They can be thought of as East and West Poles.

Magnetic Therapy works by affecting our blood. Normally the blood operates in a North Pole orientation, or under a North Pole effect. In this polarity the blood is oxygenated and its process of distributing nutrients and pulling wastes and toxins from injured tissue is made most efficient. When the body is ill or injured the polarity of the site is switched by the body to a South Pole orientation. This creates faster, excited movement meant to draw blood cells to the area for healing. The blood does not work well in a South Pole orientation. Its movement does not allow normal function and an acid state is developed, which micro-organisms, viruses and malignance thrive in.

Once the blood has been drawn to the area, the body, with the help of the Earth's magnetic field is supposed to change the polarity of the blood back to a North Pole orientation so positive activity by the blood may take place.

The problem is that with a reduced magnetic field the body can not always make this necessary conversion and the injury/illness area is left in a South Pole orientation thwarting good cell growth with its acid effect and slowing the healing process. Without blood removing wastes and toxins from injury/illness sites they are left there to fester and become unwanted bursas or arthritic tissue or bad calcification. The increase in conditions like Arthritis, Rheumatoid Arthritis, Fibromyalgia, ADD, ADHD and a multitude of cancers and other Auto-Immune system diseases have increased with the decrease of the magnetic field. Other problems are slow healing in fracture sets and longer recovery periods of disability after accidents. Another sign of this is the great increase in repetitive motion injuries in every form of business and sport. The answer in many cases is Proper Polarity Magnetic Therapy.

By applying a structured North Pole magnetic field, using high strength Neodymium magnets or a patterned North Pole pad, we can convert the polarity of the blood in the injury/illness area allowing the blood to work as it should, pulling wastes and toxins away to the kidneys and other cleansing organs, clearing a path for good cell growth aided by the nutrients the blood can now deliver. Simple and totally natural. Use a Natural field to act as a catalyst to normal blood functions. The body can now heal itself naturally. Of course if there are broken bones or vertebrae out of place the magnets will not do it alone, this is time for a good chiropractor. Magnetic Therapy is only a piece of the health pie allowing us to avoid in many cases unnatural medicines and sometimes making surgical procedures unnecessary.

Magnetic Therapy works great on many conditions and studies are coming up with more uses every day. Like the positive effects of drinking North Pole magnetized water for those with conditions like the Arthritis's, Fibromyalgia, Gout and ADHD to name a few. People are having great success but that's not a reason to avoid health professionals. After all without good diagnosis what do we treat? Magnetic Therapy works as well on Horses, Dogs and Cats as it does for people.

Apply a natural North Pole magnetic field. Convert the polarity of the blood to the North Pole orientated working polarity. Let the body heal itself. What is more natural than that?

The   Magnetic   Effect
A magnet or electromagnet produces an energy field
Each pole of a magnet produces a different effect;

North-Negative

Has a counter-clockwise rotation

Inhibits/relieves pain

Reduces inflammation

Produces an alkaline effect

Reduces symptoms

Fights infections

Supports healing

Reduces fluid retention

Increases cellular oxygen

Encourages deep restorative sleep

Produces a bright mental effect

Reduces fatty deposits

Establishes healing polarity

Stimulates melatonin production

Normalizes natural alkaline pH

South-Positive

Has a clockwise rotation

Excites/increases pain

Increases inflammation

Produces an acid effect

Intensifies symptoms

Promotes micro-organisms

Inhibits healing

Increases fluid retention

Decreases tissue oxygen

Stimulates wakefulness

Has an over-productive effect

Encourages fatty deposits

Polarity of an injury site

Stimulates body function

TREATMENT

During the initial, acutely painful stage of frozen shoulder,

rest   is   usually   advised.
Applying hot or cold packs can help.

Applying magnets

Apply two magnets on either side of the cervical vertebrae at the most painful sites. Magnetic patches can also be applied to acupuncture points over or near the site of pain. Select the points which most closely relate to the site of discomfort. **Make certain that you apply North side**

Negative to each place. The magnetic should be marked – or N or may be coloured Green (Positive will be marked + or S or red in colour).

NEUROMUSCULAR MASSAGE

This specialised form of treatment has a good record of benefits for people who have suffered a whiplash – and other – injury. However, it is not advisable to attempt to treat oneself and a visit to a certified massage therapist should not be expensive.

Spinal Degeneration/Stenosis

Spinal degeneration is usually caused by osteoarthritis and is often called *degenerative disc disease*. A development of this can lead to *spinal stenosis,* which basically means a narrowing of the spinal canal. This can be dangerous insofar as it can compress the spinal cord causing pain and/or numbness and, at its worst, can lead to paralysis. A pinched nerve might cause numbness and tingling, and nocturnal pain is not uncommon. Ligaments can thicken, bone spurs can develop, and compression fractures of the spin can occur.

Orthodox treatments consist of anti-inflammatory drugs (NSAIDs), traction in some cases, physiotherapy and an exercise programme and, as a last resort, surgery. Stretching and muscle-strengthening exercises might help reduce the pain and relieve some of the other symptoms. However, medical opinion agrees that the condition is not normally reversible.

There are, fortunately, a number of alternative treatments that have brought not only a reduction or even removal of pain but have also reversed the degenerative process.

Solutions

HOMEOPATHY

This can bring about dramatic benefits in a wide variety of ways. Not only do some of the remedies help reduce pain significantly but many of the side effects – burning, numbness, tingling, etc. – can be quickly alleviated. As always, professional help should always be sought for homeopathic remedies in order to find the most efficacious potency and remedy although it is possible to buy directly from a homeopathic supplier – some useful addresses will be given at the end of this book in Appendix C.

Lachesis particularly effective for helping when pain comes in waves across the back of the neck.

Psorinum helps with pain at night – in bed – especially where it seems to come in hammer-like blows, one after the other.

Calcarea arsenica helps reduce pain and stiffness in neck.

Silicea, where pain begins in nape of neck and quickly spreads over the head and settling behind the eyes.

Veratrum album helps when pain comes in flashes and where the neck feels so weak it becomes difficult to hold the head up normally.

Lachnantes, for pain and stiffness of the neck, sometimes feeling as if there has been a dislocation of the vertebrae.

Dulcamara, when pain moves up from nape of neck, also spreading across the shoulders

NUTRITION

Glucosamine and Chondroitin, help to prevent the degeneration of cartilage in the vertebral joints, and Chondroitin sulphate also helps reduce inflammation and pain.

Magnesium, helps improve bone mineral density – an underlying cause of spinal degeneration. Food rich sources include cashew nuts, almonds, peanuts, halibut, spinach and cereals.

Omega-3 fatty acid, deficiency is also thought to contribute to bone loss. Can be taken orally in capsule form. Food rich sources: salmon, mackerel, tuna, sardines, herring.

Vitamin A, helps prevent degeneration of the cervical spine, and also helps reduce inflammation and ensuing pain. Can be taken in capsule form, but care must be taken not to exceed 700mcg for women and 900mcg for men. Food rich sources include carrots, kale, apricots, papaya, spinach and chicken or beef liver.

VIBROFUSION

H694 Spinoflo, strongly helps connective tissue and cartilage repair. Contains the following:

Calendula officinalis 3x

Echinacea purpurea 3x

Symphytum officinale 3x

Rhododendron chrysanthum 3x

Shark and bovine ligament and cartilage 3x, 6x

Ruta graveolens 4x

Collagen, elastin 4x, 12x, 20x, 60x

Silicea 5x, 6x, 12x

Hypericum perforatum 6x

Euphrasia officinalis 6x

Aceticum acidum 6x

Arnica Montana 6x

Glycine, Alanine, Serine, Proline 6x, 12x, 20x, 30x

Formica rufa 30x

H224 Pain #1, helps relieve cervical pain.

Salix alba 3x, 6x

Selenium metallica 6x

Zincum metallicum 6x

Vitamins A, C, E 6x

Acetaminophen 6x, 12x, 30x

Ibuprofen 6x, 12x, 30x

Acetylsalicylic acid 6x, 12x, 30x

Arsenicum metallicum 6x, 12x, 30x

Arum maculatum 6x, 12x, 30x

Major nodes sarcode 6x, 12x, 30x, 60x, 100x

Mercurius vivus 30x

H88 Degenex, helps repair degenerative tissue:

Viscum album 6x, 12x, 30x, 100x

Naja tripudians 8x, 12x, 30x

Ovine glandular tissue 4x, 20x

Interferon α, ß, γ 12X, 24X, 30X

Interluken I, II, III 12x, 24x, 30x

Chapter 4

Allergy Testing and Treatment

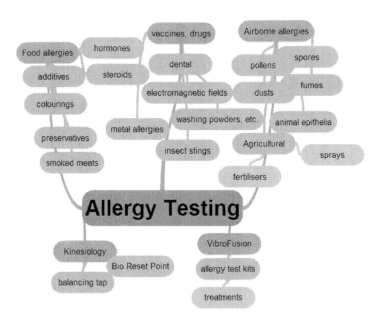

Allergy is one of the most common ailments of the modern world. It has been estimated that at least half of the entire world's population suffers from some type of allergy. Allergies can be either mild (like a skin rash or irritation)

or serious (like asthma, which kills hundreds of thousands each year).

Allergies can be subdivided into two categories:

Food allergies

Airborne allergies

Food allergies, which consist of anything – solid or liquid – which is ingested by mouth, are now suspected of underlying such major diseases as diabetes, heart disease, arthritis and several types of cancer.

Airborne allergies, or better, non-food allergies, are substances such as pollens, spores, fumes or dusts which float in the air and are inhaled into the body, or those various substances which come into direct contact with the skin and cause problems like skin ulcerations, asthma, bronchitis and emphysema – to name but a few.

Most doctors maintain that the prime cause of any kind of allergy is the *allergen* – the substance which causes the allergy. In other words, the cause of food allergy is the offending food, the cause of asthma is dust or cat hair, the cause of hay fever is pollen, and the cause of dermatitis is whatever comes into skin contact which causes an inflammatory response. The conventional approach, therefore, is that the allergen is the main problem and the cure is for the person to avoid the allergen however possible. He or she may be advised to take drugs (anti-histamines or anti-inflammatories)., or have regular injections over a period of perhaps several years.

The obvious question is, If allergens <u>cause</u> the problem why isn't everybody allergic? For many years, conventional medicine totally ignored and scoffed at the concept of allergies. More recently, however, they have concluded that it has a genetic basis – that it 'runs in families'. Even if that answer were acceptable, the question could be modified to, Why do allergies run in this particular family? Or, Why do some members of the family develop allergies while others do not?

These concepts fail to take into account that we are all unique individuals and that, rather than being humans battling against invaders from the elements, we are humans who are unable to adapt and live in harmony with our environment. To give an example, the oldest form of life on this planet is fungi. The reason it has survived since the beginning of organic time is that it has been able to adapt to whatever changes are taking place in the natural environment. I'm going to come back to the question of fungi later, because you will soon see that they have an important bearing on the subject.

Look for example, at the changes that have taken place around us in the last twenty-five years.

Food changes have taken place at many levels:

- Food growth has been interfered with chemically in many ways that are outside the awareness of most people
- Chemical fertilisers are used in place of the former methods of using natural fertilisers
- The use of chemical insecticides, herbicides, fungicides is now widespread

Natural minerals are leached from the soil and are not now replaced, and since vegetables can only contain minerals from the soil in which they are grown, it follows that many vegetables no longer contain minerals which are necessary for good health.

Added to this, animals bred for food are fed chemicals – hormones – that make them grow much faster, much leaner, and with much less waste. Not only does this make them less tasty, it also means that residues of the antibiotics and steroids injected into them find their way into us. Grass-eating animals like cows are being fed chicken meat to help provide more protein, hence the development of *mad-cow disease,* which has its human form in *Jacob-Krunzfeld Disease* that has already taken many lives.

Further up the food chain, the general use of chemicals which help preserve length of life, that give food a more 'appealing' colour, or a nicer taste, has had the effect of flooding our bodies with aggravating chemicals which can have a variety of side-effects. It has possible today – in a laboratory – to make a bar of soap absolutely irresistible. It is not stretching the imagination too far to say that if the cost of soap was cheap enough, that is what we would all be eating because the laboratory could make it taste juicier than the most succulent steak, or even strawberries and cream.

On the question of airborne allergies, think about it for a moment. Exhaust fumes from cars, toxic fumes from factories, sprays from farmers that use a variety of chemicals – and these sprays can be carried on prevailing winds for many kilometres – reach our nostrils without any difficulty, as do rains which contain toxic acid fumes from industrial factories in other countries. All of these things help weaken our immune systems.

Then there are the invisible hazards: the overhead electrical cables, which throw out a harmful electromagnetic field (VLF) which affects everything and everybody within a range of 200 metres; the harmful radiation effects from television and computer monitors, and from fluorescent lighting that most offices use; the equally harmful effects of microwave ovens that not only damage the food but also people within a range of 50 metres in all directions. And so on.

Normally the body is able to compensate for almost everything that can be thrown at it. Not only is it a miracle of creation, it is a miracle of adaptation. This is because no matter what happens outside the body, chemical compensations take place within it to bring it back into balance.

Things can go wrong, however. The last 60 years or so has seen the widespread and almost indiscriminate use of anti-biotics. These have the effect of killing off a lot of bacteria, good or bad (because not all bacteria is bad), thus interfering with the balance and allowing either or both fungi and viruses to proliferate.

One of the symptoms to follow is the development of first an intolerance and then allergy, which can be either or both related to digestion or respiration, depending on which type of fungus spreads the most: *Candida albicans* (which affects digestion) or *Aspergillus fumigatus* (which affect respiration, and cause either asthma or bronchitis).

So when we start to develop allergies we have to look carefully at all the factors involved and examine where the imbalances fall. We need to look at personal health history (especially the use of any chemical drugs like anti-biotics or steroids), genetic history, diet, lifestyle, relationships, working and recreational environment. This involves taking a comprehensive case history, followed by muscle testing.

The case history needs to include as well as the items mentioned above, a complete list of symptoms, age of symptoms and their severity. Symptoms may include any of the following:

Gastrointestinal

      inflamed, sore lips

      excessive salivation

      passing gas

      itching of roof of mouth

      air swallowing

      repeating a taste

      nausea

      vomiting

      nervous stomach

      heartburn

      indigestion

      abdominal pain

      bloating

      belching

ulcer

cramps

diarrhoea

constipation

anal itching

Skin

hives or welts

dermatitis (eczema)

adult acne

itching

burning

flushing

pallor

excessive sweating

General appearance

pale and sallow appearance

swollen face

enlarged lymph nodes

excess weight

excess thinness

Respiratory

runny nose

itching nose

nasal congestion

nasal polyps

sneezing

post-nasal discharge

nosebleed

hay fever

laryngitis

frequent clearing of throat

cough or wheeze

night cough

coughing up phlegm

asthma

difficulty breathing

bronchitis

shortness of breath

emphysema

Cardiovascular

rapid heart beat

palpitations

skipped heart beats

chest pain

ankle or calf swelling

fainting spells

flushing

chills

hot flashes

night sweats

high blood pressure

low blood pressure

Musculoskeletal

muscle spasm

muscle pain

muscle cramps

muscle weakness

neck pain

stiff neck

arthritis

rheumatism

backache

Miscellaneous conditions

anaemia

addictions (alcohol, drugs, food)

tiredness

uterine fibroids

fibrocystic breast disease

cancer

autoimmune disease

Urinary and Genital

frequent urination

painful urination

burning on irritation

urinating at night

enuresis (poor bladder control)

urgency to urinate

blood in urine

incomplete emptying

frequent urinary infections

general itching or pain

Eyes

eye pain

itching of eyes

photophobia

blurred vision

refractive changes

watering

allergic black eyes

puffy lids

red, bloodshot eyes

bags, dark circles under eyes

cataract

inflammation of iris

Ears

fluid in ears

earache

ringing in ears

vertigo

hearing loss

excessive ear wax

ear popping

flushed, red ear lobes

Nervous System and Behavioural

headache

numbness and tingling

restlessness

nervousness

jitteriness

tremor

irritability

insomnia

convulsions

anxiety

fear or panic reactions

confusion

clumsiness, poor coordination

feelings of apartness

floating sensation

amnesia

memory problems

inability to concentrate

learning disorders

minimal brain dysfunction

hyperactivity

behavioural problems

inappropriate emotional outbursts

uncontrolled anger

tension-fatigue syndrome

depression

personality changes

paranoia

hallucinations

The above is not a complete list, nor does it mean that any of the symptoms listed is caused by an allergy, as there can be other factors too. However, it does give a good guideline, especially if a person has several of the symptoms listed.

Muscle Testing

Once we are satisfied that allergy could indeed be a problem, and we have taken a good case history, we are ready to start testing, using kinesiology. Before doing the testing we are going to perform a *balancing tap*, to ensure the testing is as accurate as possible.

Balancing Tap

At the point where your collarbone meets your breastbone, or sternum, you will find a V shape at the base of your neck. He point we will be working at is about 7 cm below this V. you will probably feel a small bump on the bone there, at the point where the 2nd ribs attach to your sternum. Now imagine a circle 10 cm in diameter, centering around this *Energy Balancing Spot*. Facing the client, the testor taps around this circle several times, in a counter-clockwise direction, for about 30 seconds (about 100 taps), using two fingers together. Tap firmly but gently, and remember that fingernails can hurt.

Muscle Testing

A normal muscle test is carried out, using the deltoid muscle, arm held about 45° to the side, at shoulder level. A light pressure is placed on the arm at the wrist area, and the testee is asked to hold firm against the pressure. The muscle should remain strong at this stage. If the muscle goes weak it may indicate dehydration, in which a glass of water should be consumed by the testee before retesting.

Now that muscle testing has been carried out successfully you are ready to test against allergies. You should already have formed an opinion whether you suspect food or airborne allergy.

Under ideal conditions, you would have a sample of everything likely to have caused the allergy. You would place each substance in turn in the testee's hand, testing the deltoid muscle each time. If the arm remains strong, it is safe to assume that the substance being tested is not the offending substance, in which case you repeat the procedure with the next substance until you find a substance that causes the arm muscle to go weak. A weak muscle indicates that you have uncovered the substance causing the allergy. Please note that there may be more than one substance involved.

I said 'ideal conditions', which of course is not often the case. Particularly when dealing with airborne allergies, of which it can be any one of a hundred or more substances. It would be rare for a practitioner to have samples of each and every one of these substances, in which case testing would be difficult and probably incomplete. Even in food allergies, it could be one or more of more than a hundred foodstuffs. The difficulties here are obvious – having the sheer volume of foodstuffs on hand, plus the fact that storing food that itself may quickly deteriorate are just two.

The remedy to this is, of course, to have a comprehensive test kit containing just about kind of substance likely to cause an allergy. This is what I use, and have been using for more than 30 years with total success. Furthermore, the vials are not subject to ageing or deterioration and will last a 'lifetime'. They are light and simple to transport around wherever I go, and I get tremendous reassurance in the knowledge that wherever I am I will be able to resolve the problem if it arises.

Treatment

Okay. So now you have found the allergen. How are you going to treat it? The obvious answer is to avoid the substance, if possible. For example, if the allergen is bread – flour is one of the most common allergens – one can avoid eating bread or other foodstuffs containing flour. At least for a while. I'm not suggesting that giving up bread is simple, but it should be preferable to suffering from the allergy, which can be debilitating.

One of the most successful treatments I have found is as follows: place the substance on the navel – while lying in a supine position (on the back, facing up) – and gently tap Stomach 1 (shown on illustration below) about 75 times. Then retest the allergen again to see if the weak muscle is now strong. This procedure can be done while standing or sitting, with the allergen held in the testee's hand while testor taps ST 1.

One of the beauties of this treatment is that the client can do this him/herself whenever necessary, holding the allergen – preferably against their navel – while tapping the Stomach 1 point.

Another highly effective kinesiological treatment for allergies is what I call *Bio Reset Point*. This involves all the beginning and end points of the head.

The rationale for this treatment is this: if we are over-exposed to a particular substance – which can be food or airborne – we can, in time, become intolerant of it and it will begin to cause various symptoms to appear. These might not be noticed, or passed off lightly, but if ignored can eventually become a fully-fledged allergy, in which the symptoms become more pronounced and more severe in their intensity.

This means that during a period of intolerance, some other organ or gland is doing its best to compensate in order for the person to be able to function as close to normal as possible. When it reaches the point that compensation is no longer possible, it becomes an allergy in which all the symptoms become more debilitating.

To test if this is the case, we need to have first of all discovered the allergen. Either holding it in hand, or placing on the navel (preferable) we then place a finger on each of the points shown on the illustration until we find a point that strengthens the weak muscle. Don't forget that the allergen will have been revealed <u>because</u> it made a muscle go weak.

If we find a test point that strengthens the weak muscle, we then tap that point 75-100 times. Then retest. If the muscle no longer shows weak when retesting, it indicates that the organ or gland that had been affected is now able to resume its normal function because it has been 'reset'. A full explanation of how this works is given in Chapter 15, under the heading *Bio Reset Points*.

VibroFusion

I have already said that I use Allergy Test kits, of which full information is given in Chapter 14. What I haven't mentioned is that my normal treatment would be to give a VF remedy. There is a remedy for every allergen found.

Here's how it works: I run through a test kit of allergens. For the sake of speed, the client will hold a complete batch of maybe 20 or so vials. If the muscle then goes weak, I will test each of the twenty vials separately to narrow it down to the actual offender. If the muscle stays strong on the complete batch, I can then discard that batch and give the client another batch, and repeat the test until I find one that weakens the muscle. This way, I can test 100 vials in thirty seconds.

And it doesn't matter whether the allergy is food or airborne because there is a test kit to cover just about every eventuality. This includes a very wide range of agricultural substances – sprays, synthetic fertilisers, antifungals, etc. There is another kit which covers a wide range of pharmaceutical products, including vaccines, etc. I even have one on cosmetics, and dental substances – fillings, adhesives, etc.

Pharmaceuticals

In recent years it has become apparent that more people – including children – are becoming allergic to a wide range of pharmaceutical drugs and products, from aspirin to some anti-biotics and anti-inflammatories. Some men have become allergic to Viagra, and some women have become allergic to their partner's semen.

In fact, no matter what the substance, somebody somewhere is going to be allergic to it. Some people are allergic to life itself, and have to spend their entire life in a kind of protective tent.

There are hundreds of environmental pollutants, including new carpets, washing powders, materials used in clothing, and so on.

One of my very early patients, a Mrs Payne from Dorset, who complained of her whole body being pain-wracked – so much so that she was unable to see me so I called on her. She had to crawl to the front door to let me in because she couldn't even stand up. I tried hypnosis and homeopathy – in fact, everything that I knew at the time – without any success. Eventually, I referred her to a colleague. I heard a little later that he had discovered her problem – using kinesiology, of which I knew almost nothing at the time – and had completely cured her. The problem had been new carpeting that she had had laid down. Once the carpeting had been replaced her health returned to normal. This case was so special to me because it led me to study Applied Kinesiology with Drs George Goodheart, Sheldon Deal and others. This goes back to the 1970s.

I include in this section metal allergies. Many people have been found to be allergic to metals placed in their ear lobes – whether rings or studs. This is often caused by cheaper metals, although some people are allergic to gold, platinum or silver. The same applies to dental work carried out. People can become allergic to a wide range of materials used by dentists, including filling material, cement, anaesthetics, cavity linings, polishing paste, porcelain for crowns and, of course, some toothpastes. A wide range of these products is available in the form of a test kit, described in Appendix A.

Electromagnetic Fields

Modern society has thrown up hundreds if not thousands of electrical gadgets and instruments – like mobile telephones – which have not been in use long enough to fully understand any health risks.

However, there are some things that we do know about. Sometimes they fall in between allergies and *hypersensitivities*. One of the most common problems concerns ELF (Extreme Low Frequency) waves, which are all around us. Of course, it becomes a greater problem if we sit in front of computers for hours on end, as so many millions of people now do – either for work or educational or personal reasons.

I know of no way that is better – or even equal – to discovering allergies than muscle testing. Certainly, orthodox medicine has no comparable way. Let me give an example: I had a patient in Cambridge: a young lady in her late teens. Her father had brought her down to Dorset, where I had my practice at the time – specialising in allergies. I gave her a thorough testing and, apart from discovering that her immune system was very weak – for which I gave her a treatment – I was not able to offer anything more. Two weeks later her father phoned to say that she was even weaker, in fact so weak he was unable to bring her down to see me again. But he still had faith in me and asked me if I could call to see her. I was able to do this, and began by asking to see all the places in the house – it was a very old kind of manor house that they had recently moved in to – where she spent most of her time. The bedroom and a chair in the living room. I tested both of these places and found that each of them were directly over a water stress. I tested the whole house, in fact, and these were the only two places that had this environmental stress. We then moved her bed to another part of her bedroom, and her chair in the living room to a different part of the room. That, together with the VibroFusion remedy I had given for her immune system, brought her strength back. There was a gradual improvement each week, and within a three month period had restored her health back to what it had been. Without muscle testing, I would never have been able to discover the root problem.

To briefly give another stark case of how kinesiology enabled me to uncover a life-threatening problem, I had a patient in the Royal Household, living in the Great Park in Windsor Castle. She had a tumour in the brain. I tested her bedroom and found that a very narrow electronic beam passed through the twelve-foot thick walls and directly through the spot where she lay her head in bed. All we needed to do was move her bed to another part of the room to place her out of danger. I wasn't treating her actual cancer. What was later discovered – not through me but through officials at the castle – was that the beam emanated from a NATO air force base several miles from Windsor. The lady in question survived her cancer, through surgery and other treatments.

So, we live in a world that has a myriad of hazards and dangers. Some of us succumb to them, others survive them. But what is clear is that allergies and hypersensitivities are on the increase, and the more tools we have to combat them the better.

Chapter 5

Special Techniques

Trauma Delete

The treatment I'm about to describe is something that I have demonstrated all over the world as the most *supreme* method I know of removing pain. I have presented this in front of audiences of several thousand people, inviting *anyone* with any kind of pain to come forward and be treated.

In **almost every case I've ever had** this treatment has been successful within a minute or two. I said in Chapter 3 that I have never had a single failure. What I mean by this is that I have never had a single case in which I have not been able to at least reduce the pain to something more bearable. There have been occasions, not very many, where time has just not been sufficient for me to carry the treatment through to a total deletion and I have had to leave the patient with perhaps a little pain but very much reduced.

Many readers will know little or nothing about Myoneurology, and the subject is too broad for me to attempt to cover here. Let me just say that it is, without doubt, the most revolutionary system of techniques that I have ever learned or heard about. I personally first learned about Kinesiology in the 1970s and went on to develop several forms of kinesiology myself, including Animal Kinesiology (AnK), Sex Kinesiology (SK), Psyche Kinesiology (PK), and many others, culminating in the development of Myoneurology.

There are thousands of myoneurologists around the world, in just about every country, and the treatment I'm about to describe should only be carried out by someone professionally qualified. Make local enquiries to find one. If you want to learn more about the subject, I would suggest calling your local *Touch for Health* branch – there's one in just about every sizeable town in the Western world.

The rationale

The body is constantly expressing externally what is going on internally. Even though the cells in our body are constantly wearing out, being destroyed in a process called *catabolism* and being replaced by new cells (*anabolism*) in a never-ending process that continues from birth until death.

Until comparatively recently it was taught that all cells in the body were replaced except brain cells and myelin sheath cells. That is why, it is said, we have so many brain cells (about 100 billion) and only use a tiny percentage of them. As brain cells die, so other existing brain cells would take over their function. We have more than enough brain cells to last our whole life. Most medical schools still teach this.

However, new research indicates that this is not the case. In fact, we use **all** our brain cells most of the time. And brain cells **are** replaced in the same way as other cells. What happens in the life of a cell is fairly simple: it takes in nutrients, metabolises them, and waste by-products are formed as a result. These waste products are excreted from the cell. And over a period of time, now known to be 7 years, the whole of the brain cell is replaced. In the sense that it didn't catabalise in the same way as other cells makes no difference. The essential point is that over a period of 7 years the whole brain cell is replaced so there is nothing left of the previous cell.

Yet our memory stretches back much longer than 7 years. That alone is proof that memory resides elsewhere than in brain cells – unless each brain cell passes on memory to the new cell. This has not yet been established.

But if there is memory in the body, then that memory would contain knowledge of all injuries and trauma that had occurred within the life of that organism. Wilhelm Reich, a one-time student of Sigmund Freud, formulated a theory that memory is held in the muscles of the body, a concept he called *muscular armouring*. He postulated that the greater the past traumas the more rigid the muscles would become.

It could well be that Reich was correct, and myoneurological research would seem to confirm it. So important is this belief that probably the single most important thing a myoneurologist can do for a patient is take a new history of all previous injuries and traumas.

What I would do is hand all patients a sheet of paper with a line drawing of a human body (male or female, accordingly), and ask them to place a small x on any part of the diagram where they knew they'd had an injury throughout the whole of their lifetime. Those injuries are to include any surgery, dentistry, sprains, fractures, blows to the body, scars etc.

Sometimes, the patient's diagram would be so filled with crosses that it would be difficult to know where to start. And it probably doesn't matter where you start anyway. Each cross contains a memory that has to be dealt with. Why? Because each x represents a neuromuscular stress that is affecting the efficiency of the whole neuromuscular system.

People would come in to see me and would say, 'I have a wonderful job, a devoted wife and family, I have no financial worries, my relationship with everyone I know is great, I have a fantastic house, a new car, we go away on holiday every year and have a wonderful time. In other words, doc, my life is as smooth and fruitful as I could possibly ask for. And yet, I have this overwhelming feeling of stress hanging over me day and night. What's going on?'

Then I explain, from looking at the diagram with all the crosses on, that although the wounds and injuries from the past have all healed up, the memory of all of them is still present. *That* is what is causing the problem, I say.

The other point worth making is that the more memories a person has of past injuries and trauma, the more vulnerable he/she will be for future injuries and trauma. Their *muscular armouring* makes them clumsy, more accident prone. So that's another good reason for wanting to clear away, to delete, these traumatic memories.

Treatment

This treatment is best done in a supine position – patient lying down on his/her back. There are two test/treatments, based on whether the pain is above or below the coccyx. If it is above the coccyx we test and treat the neck; if below the coccyx, we test/treat the talus-calcaneus joint – located in the heel of the foot.

We need, for every different patient and treatment, some kind of benchmark by which we can measure progress. I use the commonly adopted one called SUDS – (Subject Units of Distress) but which I prefer to call PAS (Personal Assessment Scale). These are measures of intensity. So I would ask: how would you describe your pain on a scale of 1-10 – ten being most intense pain, one being minimum amount of pain?

If the answer is, say, 8, then we have something to measure against. If, after the treatment, we ask the same question again, and get an answer of perhaps 3, then we can assume that what've done has had a significant effect. If the answer was 7, or even 6, I would assume the treatment has had little or no effect. So that's how we use the PAS benchmark.

Test/Treatment of Pain above the Coccyx

The next thing to do is to ask the patient to place a finger, or better, 2 fingers, on the point where they feel pain. Or maybe the place represented on the diagram where they had placed an x. With the finger(s) still touching that point, we then take the patient's other arm, lift it so that it is level with the shoulder and held rigidly in position, say 'Just hold it like that' while pressing down on the arm. Not heavily, just lightly pressing down.

There are two possibilities at this point. The arm will be either as rigid as before, or it will be weaker and will not be able to resist the pressure. Either result is important, for different reasons.

If the muscle goes weak, it shows that the pain indicates an *Organic* problem, and as such cannot be ameliorated by this treatment. [This statement is not strictly true. It can be treated, but the treatment is much more complex and will not be dealt with here.]

Organic pain means there is a physiological factor involved and it would not be appropriate to remove pain (which is only a symptom) while the underlying cause is not being dealt with.

So, what we're looking for is the muscle to remain strong. Then, with patient still touching the point of pain, he/she should *extend the head* – that means that he/she should bend the head backwards. We then retest the muscle as before. If the muscle remains strong it indicates that the patient's fingers are not touching the *exact* spot of the historical trauma/injury. So we would ask the patient to move the fingers to a slightly different place and test all over again.

If, on the other hand, the muscle now goes weak,

273

we have uncovered a *Psychogenic* problem, which is what we're after. The place where the memory of the injury/trauma is stored.

To delete this memory – and the pain it brings with it – we simply put the head into *flexion*: bend it forward, while the patient maintains the fingers touching the point. Bending the head forward, putting it into flexion, means extending the range of the movement slightly more than the patient would do him/herself. Nothing vigorous, just a gentle movement, repeated perhaps 3-5 times. Bending the head forward – with both hands cupped under the head to give it support – and then lowering it gently back down. It's always best, I find, to inform the patient exactly what you intend doing and then keep to it. Never do anything you haven't told the patient has always been my policy. It takes the anxiety away.

After all this has been done, ask patient how he/she would rate it on the PAS scale. You're aiming at 1 or even zero, so under normal circumstances I wouldn't want to stop until I had achieved a total relief of pain. Occasionally, flexing the head 3-5 times is not quite sufficient and it needs to be done a couple more times.

Once you've got it down to 1 you can move on to the next point and repeat the procedure all over again. This might seem a lengthy procedure but believe me, once you know what you're doing, each stage takes only a few seconds. The whole procedure I've explained above would take me about half a minute. So I could do a whole lot of different points in half an hour.

Test/Treatment Below the Coccyx

This is a much more difficult method of testing and treating and usually requires the services of a skilled myoneurologist. The reason why this method is used is because the patient, lying supine, cannot normally reach places much below the coccyx. Therefore the practitioner has to both TP (test point) and test/treat simultaneously. The alternative to this difficult procedure is to ask the patient to sit up, if he/she is capable, and TP the place of the pain.

For testing, a finger is placed on the TP while the talus-calcaneus joint (TCJ) is jammed by striking the underside of the calcaneus bone – or heel bone – sharply with the edge of the hand. The arm is then MN tested in the normal way. There is a time-window of about 3-5 seconds between striking the calcaneus bone and testing the arm muscle. So let's just go through the procedure again:

Test the muscle – should be strong

TP the pain point – should be strong

Strike underside of the calcaneus bone

Test arm muscle – if strong, the TP is not the place of pain; if muscle goes weak, TP is correct and this point can be treated

For treating, finger remains on the same TP while the therapist holds the heel firmly and, with a sharp tug, creates what we call a gap in the TCJ. The arm muscle is then tested in the same way as before. The expert myoneurologist can tell when this has been achieved successfully and in some cases this might have to be repeated several times before success is achieved. So again, let's review the procedure:

Therapist cradles the heel in palm of hand

Tugs sharply on calcaneus bone

Tests arm muscle – should be strong

Strikes sharply on underside of calcaneus bone

Tests the arm muscle – if treatment is successfully completed should be strong, if arm muscle goes weak means the 'gapping' has not been successful

The corollary of all this is that if difficulty is experienced testing and/or treating the TCJ then try testing/treating pain points below the coccyx using the head flexion/extension method. It will work just as efficiently except that the patient might have some difficult TPing the pain point. In which case it might be possible for the testor to TP the pain point.

Another possibility is for a *surrogate* – third person – to TP the pain point while at the same time placing a hand on the shoulder or thigh of the testee. The testor can then proceed to test and treat as though the testee were TPing the point.

Bio Reset Point

Homeostasis is a term that was coined by Walter Cannon from two Greek words meaning *to remain the same*. In the human body it has come to mean the body's ability to adjust the *internal* environment within tolerable limits in order to maintain a stable condition.

For example,

- the skeletal muscles can shiver to produce heat if body temperature drops too low

- sweating helps cool the body, with the use of evaporation, if the body temperature gets too high

- the pancreas produces insulin if too much sugar enters the blood; it also produces glucagons if the blood sugar level drops too low

- the kidneys remove urea and adjust the concentrations of water and mineral ions

277

The concept is that different organs, different systems in the human body, have a set point at which they function optimally.

The set point is regulated by the hypothalamus gland – the body's master gland – which sets upper and lower tolerance levels. These are probably determined at a genetic level before birth but undergo many adjustments after birth. The internal environment is influenced by the external environment. Thus the Eskimo is able to tolerate much lower temperatures than the Kalahari bushman, while the bushman is able to endure much higher temperatures than the Eskimo.

It's what we get used to.

The problem is that many of us get used to things that are not actually good for us. If we keep ingesting sugar, for example, we force the pancreas to produce more and more insulin in order to maintain blood-sugar equilibrium. Two things can happen here: the pancreas over-produces insulin, takes too much sugar out of the blood, and sparks off a stream of hypoglycaemic symptoms – drowsiness, fatigue, irritability, inability to concentrate, memory dysfunction and so on; if the pancreas goes on over-producing, eventually it becomes exhausted, at which point it is unable to produce *sufficient* insulin and diabetes mellitus begins to set in.

This happens because the normal limits and

tolerances of homeostasis have been exceeded. If we are able to **reset** those limits, then the person will not present with hypoglycaemic symptoms *unless* he exceeds the new limits. It could be argued that by resetting the limits we are encouraging the person to consume more of the offending substance. It could equally be argued that if the person is going to do that anyway, all we are doing is ensuring he is still able to function normally while doing so.

If we apply the same principle to pain, it's well known that we all have what is called a 'pain threshold'. Some people's threshold is higher than others, meaning that they are able to withstand pain to a greater degree. If we are able to reset the Set Point (SP), or limits, we are going to enable a person to withstand a higher level of pain.

That has to be reasonable, doesn't it?

The answer to that is yes and no. If, for example, a person has a crippling illness that is causing intense pain, then anything we can do – without involving chemical drugs – is surely desirable. On the other hand, if a footballer, for example, has receiving a damaging kick on the foot or leg and the coach wants him to play on – using one of those anaesthetic sprays to deaden the pain – then the player runs the risk of further damaging the foot or leg. In such a case, the use of a spray – or the myoneurological equivalent, Homeostatic Set Point – would not be good.

So it's all relative. If ingesting more sugar – or any other food – is going to be harmful to the person, taking everything into consideration, then raising the SP is not a good idea. But if raising the SP is actually going to be beneficial, then it is a good idea. So everything should be evaluated and determined on an individual basis.

In *most* cases, it will be seen to be beneficial. After all, raising the SP is not the same thing as saying the person can have as much sugar as he/she wants no matter how much harm it will ultimately cause. Because the body still has *ultimate* limits and tolerances – it's just that these have been raised a little to enable the person to function better.

Here's how we're going to be able to change the tolerance levels of our pain. To do so, we are going to use all the *acupuncture head points* in which acupuncture channels or meridians start or end on the head.

We begin by asking the patient to place a finger on the point in the body where pain is felt most acutely. If we test the muscle in the other arm (arm held out level with shoulder to the side) by pressing down lightly, it should go weak. This indicates that we have the right point. If the muscle stays strong, ask patient to move finger slightly and retest. Keep doing this until a point is found that weakens the muscle being tested.

Then the testor (person doing the testing) places a finger on each of the acupuncture head points in turn while testee (person being tested) keeps finger on pain point) until a point is found that *strengthens* the arm muscle. That indicates that a meridian has been found that will raise the Set Point. Then testor simply taps that head point about 50-75 times while testee keeps finger on pain point.

To find out if you've accomplished anything, you retest the pain point again – on its own – and if the muscle now tests *strong* it indicates that you have raised the SP. Whether you've changed it enough depends on how the patient feels about the pain. Has it gone? Is it reduced? Should we try to reduce it some more? These are questions you can ask.

If we apply the same principle to weight, it's well established that we all have what is called a 'weight threshold'. This threshold does not remain constant throughout our lifetime. It will vary according to various factors. For example, as infants we start to gain weight rapidly as our body goes through the growing cycles, and the appestat regulates the weight threshold accordingly. A woman going through pregnancy gains weight, and again the appestat regulates. If we abuse our diet – like consuming excessive carbohydrates over a prolonged period – then the appestat is likely to reset itself at a higher level to allow the body to accept the additional weight.

What happens when we go on a diet is that we lose weight and the appestat has to keep adjusting downwards. The problem is that we have a *memory* of all the weights and appestat set points throughout our life. Losing weight, in itself, does not reset the appestat, so it is inevitable that weight is likely to revert back to what it was before starting the diet – very often with a little added on as a precaution against future loss. It does this because the brain has come to believe that that weight is what it should be.

So diet does not work **because it does not reset the appestat**.

We begin by asking the person to place a finger on the umbilicus (navel). If we test the muscle in the other arm (arm held out level with shoulder to the side) by pressing down lightly, it should be strong. We then ask testee (person being tested) to turn head to the left and retest the muscle. If the muscle now goes weak it indicates that we have the right point. If the muscle stays strong, ask patient to move finger slightly and retest. Keep doing this until a point is found – in the area of the umbilicus – that weakens the muscle being tested – when the head is turned to the left.

Then the testor (person doing the testing) places a finger on each of the acupuncture head points (listed above) in turn, while testee keeps finger on umbilicus, until a point is found that *strengthens* the previously weak arm muscle. That indicates that a meridian has been found that will change the Set Point beneficially. Then testor simply taps that head point about 50-75 times while testee keeps finger on umbilicus.

To find out if you've accomplished anything, you retest the umbilicus again – on its own, but with head turned to left – and if the muscle now tests *strong* it indicates that you have changed the SP.

Ileocecal/Houston Valve

Although I would like to outline this treatment here, I have decided it is too complex to be attempted by a lay person, so would urge you to find a good, local myoneurologist or kinesiologist who is familiar with the technique. The test and treatment, completely painless, is so fast to perform and effective, that it will be well worth seeking out a myoneurologist who can help.

This refers to all pain that is related to the gastrointestinal tract, constipation or other colon-related condition (persistent diarrhoea, Crohn's disease, irritable bowel syndrome, and so on).

The Test

We start by finding a strong indicator muscle [tests deltoid]. Okay, now we're going to challenge that by finding this point – we feel for the iliac fossa, which is the bony protuberance of the pelvis, then we move two inches medial - towards the centre of the body – and two inches inferior – down – which gives us this point, which is called McBurney's Point. If we push very lightly – keeping our fingertip on the McBurney Point – towards the contralateral shoulder – which is always going to be her left shoulder – and retest the muscle, and look … the muscle has gone weak. That indicates an open ICV syndrome. If I push away from the contralateral shoulder and the muscle goes weak, it indicates a closed ICV syndrome.

Treatment

Okay, the ICV is held in position and regulated by four sets of muscles. So the McBurney Point was for testing, now for treatment you have to go to the ICV point itself [placing two fingers lightly over the point, which is the lower end of the caecum on the right side of the person's abdomen]. First part of the treatment is to locate the weak muscle: one of the four muscles is usually going to be weak, the other three muscles are usually going to be strong. If more than one of the four muscles goes weak, then prioritise to find which muscle to treat first. [to prioritise, place the tip of the middle finger against the first crease on the inside of the thumb – on the hand not being used to locate the ICV – and push down lightly on the indicator muscle] So let's just do this again, to make sure you're following me: I always think of it in terms of North – towards the head – South – towards the feet – East – towards left side – and West – towards the right side – directions. So with the fingers lightly pressing in a northerly direction test the muscle. Note if weak or strong, remember you're looking for a weak muscle. Then lightly press in a southerly direction and test the muscle, noting whether weak or strong. Repeat this pressing lightly in easterly and westerly directions. At the end of this testing, which takes less than 5 seconds, you will normally find one weak muscle and three strong muscles. Okay, so if we find that pressing in a northerly direction shows a weak muscle the treatment is to press and *stretch* the same place in the opposite direction - southerly. But in a special way.

What I want the patient to do is to take three deep breaths – when I tell you to start – and while you are inspiring draw both legs together up towards your chest. Then as you expire, or exhale, straighten your legs out and lower them gently. And while you're exhaling and lowering your legs, I shall be lightly pressing on the ICV point in a southerly direction. And we're going to do this three times. So let's do it. [treatment carried out] Good.

Now we want to find out if we've fixed the problem, so we go back to the McBurney Point and retest all over again. See what's happened? Where the muscle went weak before we did the treatment it's now very strong. Which indicates that we've accomplished something. The real test will come, of course, when the patient is able to see if the diarrhoea she's been experiencing has now stopped.

What would happen if the McBurney Point test still went weak? Would that mean the treatment hasn't worked?

It might mean that, but it also might mean that we need to repeat the treatment we just gave maybe once or twice. Sometimes three times just isn't quite enough. Then we might get a strong muscle. If the muscle is still weak, we can go the Houston Valve test point, which is on the left side of the body, exactly the same, two inches medial from the iliac fossa and two inches inferior. Then test. In the case just illustated, the point tests strong. If it had gone weak, we would treat in exactly the same as for the ICV, only on the left side of the abdomen. So we would go down here to a point that corresponds to the Houston Valve, pressing lightly in the North, South, East and West directions, the same as for the ICV.

What actually causes either the ICV or the Houston valve to dysfunction?

It's not enough just to fix a problem, though that is

what so many practitioners. Hyperacidity or hyperalkalinity are two main causes. To get down to even more fundamental causes we have to go to the Enteric Nervous System – the ENS – because that controls everything that happens in the alimentary canal. But the ENS itself acts in response to what is happening somewhere along its length – which, as we know, can be anywhere from the mouth to the anus. We now know that something called the ileal brake slows down the peristaltic action to prevent undigested fats from passing through the ICV into the ascending colon. It does this because undigested fats encourage the growth of the so-called *unfriendly bacteria* – the types that can cause infection (and worse) within the colon. So we can say that undigested fats cause a closed ICV. The most common fat that causes this is *hydrogenated fat*.

The open ICV is caused by the presence of unabsorbed sugar, which provides sustenance and energy for the unfriendly bacteria. The probable main reason for the sugar being present is Insulin Resistance – sometimes called Insulin Insensitivity. The two main causes of Insulin Resistance are the production of excess cortisol – made in the adrenal glands – usually as a result of excessive stress, or too much oestradiol – the female sex hormone, produced in small amounts in the adrenals glands of the male. So because ingested sugar cannot be transported into cells that need it, it floats about in the bloodstream, like lost lambs in a snowstorm. Much of it will be excreted through the kidneys and urine and any other will find its way into the lumen of the small intestine.

The ICV is affected by the *content* of the colon and in particular, by the pH. I said earlier that the ascending colon was very slightly alkaline, whereas the last part of the small intestine is slightly acidic. So bacteria like to live in the ascending and transverse colon, and most of it is fairly friendly. But the warm, damp environment also attracts several different types of parasites, and they can create valvular problems. It is also true to say that anything that happens anywhere along the alimentary canal can affect any other part of it.

A good example of this is the diaphragm, up here in the chest. That has a kind of flap that allows food to pass through it in a downwards direction but normally closes to prevent anything travelling in the opposite direction. If it wasn't able to do this, every time you were in an upside-down position the whole contents of your stomach would reflux up into your mouth. Now it's true that this does sometimes happen, usually as a result of fermentation in the stomach creating a large volume of gas which puts pressure on the oesophageal sphincter causing it to open up. If it does that, it's showing you have a problem with the diaphragm.

Self Destruct – Syndrome Y

After I developed my concept and treatment of Self Destruct I later called it *Syndrome Y*, basically because I found it to be such a common and widespread problem.

When I first stumbled on this as a treatment technique (more than 30 years ago) I knew it worked but I didn't know how or why. Now I do know, and I've already touched upon it earlier when I mentioned John Diamond's test.

Because the place we go to, where we put our hand when myoneurologically testing for self-destruct – directly over the solar plexus – is directly over the Third Brain – the Enteric Nervous System – an enormous network of nerves that has an intelligence quite distinct from the first Brain – the one in our head.

It is one of the main reasons that prevents people from getting better.

So the concept is that a person seems to obey some hidden, internal command that works against the person's best interests. Now, the really big question is, Why would a person go against their own best interests?

Remember, nothing happens by accident. There is a compelling reason behind every act, every behaviour we have.

I believe that all self-destruct commands come about because of something that was said to us at an earlier time in our life. If you think back, for a moment, try to recall if any of these commands have been given to you in the past:

'Shut up'

'You're just a child'

'You're nothing'

'You're stupid'

'Grow up'

'You'll never amount to anything'

'You're a bad person'

'You're not a nice person'

'You can never do anything properly'

'You're dumb'

'You don't know anything'

'You're worthless'

'You're useless'

'You can never remember anything'

'You'll never please anybody'

'You'll grow up to be fat and lazy'

and so on.

There are two things about these commands:

1. they all (except for the first one I gave you) start with the word 'you' or 'you're' (you are)

2. because they are words, they are received by that part of the brain that deals with speech sensory input, which is called *Wernicke's area* [see above diagram]. The *arcuate fasciculus*, while appearing to join the Wernicke's area with the Broca's area is, in fact, a neural pathway that joins the *temporoparietal junction* with the frontal cortex of the brain.

It's hard to believe, but this is the point we've always used for testing the hypothalamus. We knew the hypothalamus controlled the limbic brain, which is responsible for memory and emotions. Now, we know it's associated with how we deal with things said to us – and the emotional tag that we put on these words. It all comes together, doesn't it! This opens up a whole new understanding of why so many of the treatments we've been using work so well.

Now let's think of the significance of this. The negative commands are being picked up by the brain's speech sensory centre, Wernicke's area, and all the commands – from another person, who may be parent,

291

sibling, teacher, peer or other – start with the word **you,** **you're** or **you'll** – you will.

In the past, haven't we always thought in terms of I?

'I am nothing'

'I am stupid'

'I should grow up'

'I'll never amount to anything'

'I'm not a nice person'

and so on.

In reality, the negative command was given in the 'you' form and these repetitive negative commands, received in the Wernicke's area, are recorded in the limbic brain. Because they are *hurtful* at the time, they are imbued with emotions which make them stick.

One-off negative commands might hurt a little at the time but are usually forgotten or shrugged off. It is the repetition of these negative commands – particularly if they are picked up by others and repeated (forming a reinforcement) – that then create **lesions** in the speech motor centre – *Broca's area.* [see last diagram]

It is this area which activates or inhibits action. And this position is at a level of the hypothalmic test point, but in front of the ear instead of behind it. If you feel around, and do it gently because the area is quite tender or sensitive, you'll find a slight niche.

So now we know a bit more than we knew before, so we are ready to start doing some testing. And the key to testing is finding the *exact wording* of the original negative command that created the lesion in the first place. This is very different from John Diamond's original treatment we used to give for self-destruct: RNA tissue and Rose water. Well, that used to clear things up for some people, but it didn't work for everyone and it didn't always last.

You see, when a person is on self-destruct course, they do all the things that will prevent them from overcoming their problem or making progress:

- ◎they'll eat the wrong foods (do we know anybody like this?) A negative command might have been: 'You'll always be fat'.
- ◎they use the wrong lighting (maybe sit struggling to read when it's already got quite dim, but they won't put on a light) A negative command: 'You'll never be able to see things clearly'.
- they always have the sound turned down too low on the radio or TV A negative command: 'You never listen to what I say'.
- they choose the wrong doctor and present with the wrong disorder (normally, both doctor and patient will presume that the patient wants to get well, and this is not always the case) A negative command:

'You'll never get better'.

- they make bad students, not because they're not intelligent but because they don't make any effort. A negative command: 'You'll never learn'.

I could go on and on, but these example make it clear enough because I'm sure that every one of us know people to whom these cases apply.

So, let's do the test devised by Dr John diamond:

1.   Test for self-destruct: Patient places right hand on solar plexus (bottom of hand resting on umbilicus) – test muscle. Should be strong. Removes hand. Testor places hand on solar plexus and tests – should be strong. Patient then places right hand on top of testor's hand, test – if strong then OK, if weak, indicates Self-Destruct.

2.   If we have a self-destruct, we proceed as follows: begin by asking a person if they have any knowledge of a negative command. They might know, or it might have been buried beneath all kinds of other debris piled on top. But if they know, it's a big help, because you can test them on it. If they don't know, ask them which area of their life is giving them problems, then try going through a variety of negative commands, trying to seek the appropriate one. Remember, you have to find the exact words that caused the lesion.

3.   To test, ask the patient to say the words –

aloud or silently, depending on their choice (they might not wish to reveal their hidden secret) – while they turn their eyes level with their ears to the left. This eye movement now takes them to the auditory centre (Wernicke's area) of the left brain, which is responsible for learning and remembering functions. Remember that you have to start each negative command with 'You' or 'You're' or 'You'll? And not with 'I', because that is how they received the command in the first place. In addition, they must STP – Subjective Test Point – the Wernicke's area on left side because that's the side in which, allegedly, memory is stored. If you get a weak muscle you can proceed to next step. If muscle is strong, it means you have not yet got the exact words you need.

4. We can now go to the Pre-motor cortex on the left side.

STP with eyes turned towards ears left. Test. If muscle goes weak, this is confirmation that we have now found the negative command or phrase that the brain is converting to self-destruct. If we do not get a weak muscle on both of these tests we can conclude that we have not found the correct negative command and must start again.

5. To test for treatment, we retest exactly as before, except eyes will be directing horizontally

right. The previously weak muscle should now be strong.

The treatment I developed is in two phases: inhale deeply with eyes closed but still directed towards the right ear, while therapist places a finger gently on SI 19, pushing very lightly in a forward direction. Then exhale, lifting finger during exhalation. Repeat 3-5 times.

Retest as before, STPing the Wernicke's area on the left side while repeating the negative command. The muscle should now be strong if the negative command has been negated. If the muscle goes weak, may need to repeat treatment phase from 3 to 5 more times. Then retest.

The ultimate retest is the Self-Destruct test, as outlined above. If muscle is now strong, indicates that the negative command is no longer adversely affecting patient, who is no longer on a self-destruct course. If the muscle goes weak, it means there might be another negative command which needs uncovering and treating.

Written Self-Destruct

This is completely new stuff. Sometimes, not as uncommon as one might think, the self-destruct course has been implanted, not by a negative command, but by something written. It could have been in the form of a letter or note, in which the patient is condemned. The guilt is immaterial. For example, someone could have written a note saying:

'You are a crook'

'You are a cheat'

'You're a wife-beater'

or whatever. As I said, it doesn't matter whether the condemnation is true or not. It doesn't matter whether the person _is_ a crook, or a cheat, or a wife-beater. We're not here to sit in moral judgement – or any other kind of judgement, for that matter. If we do sit in judgement, then we're in the wrong job. Get out now, while there's still time.

Or writing may have been scrawled on patient's door, or window, or somewhere where it can be seen by others.

PERVERT

WIFE-BEATER

POOF

Or whatever. The net effect is the same.

In the same way that we have areas that deal with speech (auditory) – Wernicke's area and Broca's area – we also have areas that deal with written (visual) information. The _inferotemporal cortex_ is the visual association equivalent to Wernicke's area. The _angular gyrus_ is responsible for converting the written word to the spoken word. Have you noticed that when we read we also speak to ourselves? Some people even speak aloud – more of a mutter – while they're reading. Others just mouth the words silently. From there, the angular gyrus, the information is conveyed to the pre-motor cortex and the Broca's area. (Patients with angular gyrus syndrome may be a precursor to Alzheimer's disease.)

The complication of all this is that the patient might be on a self-destruct course because of something written rather than the negative command we've been speaking of. So we need to try and ascertain that. They might be able to tell you. Or you can muscle test, while asking:

'Does your problem relate to something *said* to you in the past?'

'Does your problem relate to something *written* to or about you in the past?'

The answer should come in the form of a strong muscle (meaning yes). A weak muscle is a 'no' indication.

The test is much the same as before, once you believe you have the exact quotation. Visual (written) condemnations are usually much more vivid in the mind of the patient, and there is a good chance s/he will be able to tell you exactly what was written. Part of the reason for this is that it would almost certainly have come later in life than the spoken command.

1.   Having written the offending words down on paper, let the patient see the paper while STPing the infero-temporal cortex point. Eyes should be looking left, obliquely up. Test the muscle. If strong, you might have the wrong words written down. If weak, proceed.

2.   Still looking obliquely up to left, STPing the angular gyrus on left side. If muscle weak, confirmation that you have the correct quotation. If strong, change words and start again.

Treatment is much the same as before, with only the following changes:

STP the Pre-motor cortex on right side, eyes looking obliquely up to right, eyes closed. While inhaling, therapist places thumb gently on SI 19, pushing very lightly in the direction of Ba Hui – Du 20. Lift finger when exhaling. Repeat 3-5 times.

Retest, holding the paper up for patient to read, while sTPing the infero-temporal cortex. If muscle now strong, means problem overcome.

To confirm this, do self-destruct test again. Muscle should now be strong throughout.

Kinesthetic Self Destruct

Now we come to the biggest mind-blower you can

imagine. Have you ever wondered why it is that kids who get abused frequently turn out to be abusers themselves in later life? I think we all know that they do, but why?

Why is it that women, or girls, who get sexually abused – rape, incest, whatever – often go through the rest of their life fearing sexual contact – sometimes even fearing the opposite sex? And, of course, to this list we can add victims of wife-beating.

You should have guessed by now that the simple answer is once they have had the experience – whether sexual or violence (and often the two go together) – they have pressed the Self-Destruct button. Not consciously. After the event, they don't sit down one day and say, 'As soon as I get the chance, I'm gonna do this to someone else.' It's done at a psycho-neurological level.

To be technical, it is done at a combined Sensorisomatic/Hypothalmic level.

The Second Somatic Sensory area (called SII) occupies the under-surface of the *parietal operculum*. It corresponds to Brodmann's area 3, which is immediately adjacent and inferior to the Pre-motor cortex.

The Pre-motor Cortex contains about 30,000 pyramidal cells known as Giant Betz cells, which make up axons. These are the largest axons in diameter in the body, and can be more than 30 cm in length. They are myelinated – encased within a sheath – and are highly specialised for conducting information. Lesions here may lead to Parkinson's disease. But what's important for us is that the length and proximity to SII of these Betz cells enables them to pick up sensory information, which it quickly transports to the hypothalamus, where it creates an emotional tag.

One bad violent sexual experience can be sufficient to trigger off a Self-Destruct reaction, like a phobia. Repeated experiences reinforce the Self-Destruct over and over. And I want to point out that Self-Destruct is not what it sounds like. It is, in fact, a defensive mechanism, designed to help the victim avoid another nasty experience, although it is not always within their ability to avoid.

Testing

Whatever the earlier experience is, because it involves violence, it will nearly always be remembered by the victim. It might be difficult for them to bring themselves to think and talk about it, but you need to try and get them to reveal their painful experience. Once you know that, STP the point immediately below the Pre-motor Cortex on the left side and test, while the patient is thinking or vocalising their experience, and while they are looking obliquely down to the left. If this is creating a Self-Destruct reaction, muscle will go weak. Sometimes you can also do this by STPing the left hypothalamus point instead of the SII point. So, if one fails, try the other. The reason there can be a variance seems to be the depth and pain created by the experience.

Treating

STP the right Pre-motor Cortex point while the patient is experiencing the event – if it is too painful, ask them to try and observe it happening to them as if on a TV screen, so they are not actually experiencing it themselves – with closed eyes looking obliquely down to the right. As person inhales, therapist places fingers lightly on SI 19 and gently pushes in the direction of the *mental protuberance* – tip of the jaw. Lift finger during exhalation. Repeat this 3-5 times.

Retest, as before: thinking of painful experience while STPing the SII point or hypothalamus on left side, and looking obliquely down to the left. If treatment successful, muscle will now be strong.

Ultimate test is to repeat the Self-Destruct test once more. Should be strong throughout..

Glycaemic Test

The following myoneurological tests can be useful indicators but should not be taken alone to determine blood sugar problems. Always follow them up with a responsible glucose tolerance test, conducted by a qualified health care professional. Remember that we are dealing with a potential life-threatening condition here.

The simple tests are as follows.

1. patient lies supine (on back) on treatment table

2. patient raises left leg about 45°. Testor places hand on ankle region and gently presses down while patient *resists*. Muscle should be strong.

3. patient now bends right leg, with foot resting on table top. Testor again presses down on the left leg. If muscle is strong it indicates that there is not a hypoglycaemic problem. If muscle tests weak it indicates that there *could* be a problem of hypoglycaemia.

4. Repeat this process, using the right leg raised 45°, first with left leg kept straight on the treatment table, then with left leg bent with foot firmly on table top. If the muscle goes weak on the second test, it could indicate that there is a hyperglycaemic condition. To reiterate, this can only be confirmed by an appropriate glucose tolerance test, to be carried out by a suitably qualified health care professional.

In either case, in the interests of the patient, their doctor should be informed or consulted as to the suspicion of a sugar problem.

Temporal Tapping

A technique aimed at reprogramming specific parts of the brain by stimulating the neuropathways of the brain. By tapping the arc from the front of the ear to the rear of the ear while at the same time saying an affirmation of how you want to change a core belief. And it's important to remember that both sides are different in the sense when you tap on the right side of the head the affirmation should be a positive one while tapping on the left side of the head should be accompanied by a double-negative affirmation. So for example, you tap on the right side and might affirm 'My prostate is free of pain' or tap on the left side and affirm 'I no longer suffer from pain in my prostate'. I'm using prostate here but the same could apply to any part of the body. So the affirmation becomes the *implant* which, after a continuous series of repeats eventually becomes a *linchpin* within a part of the brain and replaces what was having previously having a negative effect on your mind and behaviour.

Temporal tapping is a technique for reprogramming your brain. It works by stimulating the receptors and neuropathways ways responsible for hanging onto our core beliefs, and by tapping this location while intending the belief we want, we can 'update our brain's operating system.'

You tap in a half-circle on the side of your head (around your ear from your –temple down to next to your earlobe) You tap while saying an affirmation phrase. I start on the right side first and go from the front to the back and then the left side from the front to the back.

If right-handed, when doing the right ear, say a positively-worded phrase such as 'I am prosperous.' When doing the left ear, use a double negative phrases such as 'I no longer worry about money.'

The reason for this is that the left brain processes double negatives things better, the right brain processes the positive better. In addition when you repeat a positive affirmation so many times after a while your brain starts to tune it out with really anchoring in as a new belief. The double negative allows your brain to process the same info but stated a little differently. Note: This is switched in left-handed people, right=neg, left=pos.)

Mitral Valve Prolapse

There are four heart valves: the aortic, pulmonary, tricuspid and mitral. The mitral valve connects the left ventricle of the heart to the left atrium. When it is open it allows blood to flow into the aorta to supply the rest of the body. If the orifice of the mitral valve has narrowed, thus reducing the flow of blood, it's called a mitral valve stenosis. If the valve is not shutting completely it is called a mitral valve prolapse, and when this prolapse allows some of the blood to leak back into the heart, it's called a mitral valve regurgitation. Either of these conditions reduces the efficiency of the heart, reduces blood circulation, and lowers endurance. That can cause fatigue, breathlessness, and obviously limits any athletic participation. About 15% of females over the age of 40 have MVP, probably without knowing it.

A diagonal crease in the ear lobe might arouse suspicion and would be worth checking out myoneurologically. It was already known that chronic circulation disorder caused the vascular bed of the earlobe to collapse, causing a visible diagonal crease in the earlobe to appear. The Mayo Clinic announced that out of 191 patients complaining of chest pain – who also had bilateral creases in their earlobes – 90% had a heart attack. Conversely, in 191 patients who complained of chest pains but did not have a creased earlobe, 90% did not go on to have a heart problem (Pearson *et al*, 1982).

To check with MN, go to test point (TP) CV (Ren) 14, known in some parts of China as the *death point*. This should test strong. Now 2-point Ren 14 with SI 19. A strong muscle means there is no mitral valve prolapse. A weak muscle would indicate that there is a *masked* MVP. Another way to check is by 2-pointing the tricuspid valve

– TP is over the xyphoid process – and the mitral valve – TP is under the left nipple. Weak muscle indicates a MVP.

Treatment

Myoneurology

Place two fingers lightly on Ren 14 and on UB 15 15 – either side of T5 –

simultaneously and hold them there for five inspirations/expirations of patient.

Retest by 2-pointing Ren 14 with SI 19. If muscle now strong, indicates prolapse has been successfully treated.

Nutritional

Magnesium – 100mg three times daily for one week

Thiamine (B1) – 250 mg once daily for one week

Pyridoxine (B6) – 50mg once daily for one week

Co-enzyme Q110 – 100mg once daily for one week

L-Carnitine – 500mg once daily for one week

Herbal

Kava – 100mg once daily for one week

Valerian – 10ml of tincture once daily for one wee

Addictions

There's a side to addictions that most people don't know. So, it doesn't really matter what the addiction is. It could be cigarettes or drugs or coffee .... or even chocolate. What is important to note is that addictions are related to anxieties. So if we want to help a person get over their addiction we have to treat their anxiety because that anxiety is actually causing the addiction. Usually, if you ask an addict why they take whatever it is they're addicted to, 99% of them will say, 'Because it makes me relax.' They've given you the answer right there. They take their substance, whatever it is, because it helps relieve their anxiety. So, conversely, if you can treat their anxiety it will help them to get rid of their addiction.

Let me give you an example. Heroine is regarded as being a highly addictive substance. Now in the UK – this isn't true for all countries – but in the UK it is perfectly legal to give heroine for pain relief in cases where the pain levels are extremely high, as in terminally ill cancer cases. Now this isn't the same in the USA, where it is not legal even in such cases. But this is the interesting part: in those cases where heroine is administered to help relieve chronic pain, when the pain has gone – let's say when the patient has been cured so they no longer need the heroine – ceasing taking the heroine does not present a problem for them. If they had been taking the same heroine for recreational purposes, if they suddenly stopped they'd go *cold turkey*. They'd go crazy. But if they've been taking heroine for pain purposes and they stop, no problem at all.

What this is saying is that the heroine creates a psychological dependence for the junkie rather than a chemical dependence. Yet for the cancer sufferer there is no dependence on the substance, either psychologically or chemically. You can prove chemically that a person who quits smoking will show no chemical signs in the body within 48-72 hours. Yet they might crave tobacco a year later. In other words, they have a psychological dependence on tobacco, not chemical. And this is as true of coffee or chocolate or whatever the addiction is. So the chemical dependence is very short-lived and what carries on is a psychological dependence.

If that is the case, it has to be treatable. And it doesn't really matter whether the addict is aware that he is really satisfying this anxiety or not. So what I'm saying is that 99% of all addictive substances have a tranquillising effect on the body, and the addiction can also create a psychological reversal which at some stage can turn into a powerful self-destructive process. That's when the person can no longer help themselves. That is quite obviously the time when they need help. And we now have an excellent way of treating this.

Appendix A

Test/Treatment Kit Compendium

Guidelines for the use of

Test kits

1. Designed to be used with kinesiology or Vega testing machines. Vial should be held in hand, arm stretched level with shoulder, to side of body. Testor presses down lightly on arm. If muscle weakens, indicates that the testee may have a problem consistent with agent represented in vial.

2. Vials designated as **remedies** should be held in hand, as before, but tested against a muscle which is already weak. If muscle becomes stronger, indicates that remedy may be suitable for treatment.

3. Any weak muscle brought about testing against a vial can also be used to test against any other

treatment. For example: Patient tests strong with normal test. Holds vial for Mercury (HH70, vial #56), which now causes the muscle to go weak. This indicates that the testee has a mercury overload, which can go on to cause a variety of problems in many parts of the body. Testee can be tested (still holding vial #56) with any number of other agents – herbal, nutritional, homeopathic, etc. to see if any of them will help. Anything likely to help will cause the previously weak muscle to now go strong.

4. We have remedies for all Test Kits, which can be ordered as a complete Remedy Kit, or as individual remedy vials (minimum of 6 individual vials for one order), or as remedy tablets (each sealed tub containing at least 90 tablets).

5. **Contents of vials should not be consumed.**

6. If in doubt, always consult a health care professional.

7. These tests are not designed to be a direct substitute for other, orthodox tests. They may imply indications that can then be tested in other ways. It is always advisable to test for any implied condition in as many ways as possible, in order to confirm.

The following gives a rounded picture of the range of test

kits available, together with prices. For a comprehensive list, or any other queries, please contact us at: vibrofusion@gmx.com

The following gives a rounded picture of the range of test kits available, together with prices. For a comprehensive list, or any other queries, please contact us at: vibrofusion@gmx.com

VF 1   **Virus/Bacterial/Fungal** – 100 vials

VF 2   **Food Allergies #1**

Meats, Fish, Seafood, Dairy, Nuts, Oils,

Drinks, Sweeteners – 100 vials

VF 3   **Food Allergens #2**

Fruit, Vegetables – 100 vials

VF 4   **Non-Food Allergens** – 100 vials

VF 5   **Blood Chemistry** – 50 vials

VF 6   **Vitamins/Minerals** – 100 vials

VF 7   **Food Additives #1**

Colourings, Preservatives, Sweeteners – 100 vials

VF 8   **Food Additives #2**

Anti-oxidants, Emulsifiers, Thickening agents,

Flavour Enhancers, Miscellaneous – 100 vials

VF 9 **Pharmaceutical Burden** – 100 vials

VF 10 **Environmental Pollutants** – 100 vials

VF 11 **Vaccination** – 18 vials

VF 12 **Bacteria** – 100 vials

VF 13 **Viruses** – 100 vials

VF 14 **Fungi/Mycoses** – 87 vials

VF 15 **Parasites** – 100 vials

VF 16 **Urine Analysis/ Pregnancy Test,**

Best Therapy Test/Prognosis/Localisation – 50 vials

VF 17 **Hormones** – 50 vials

VF 18 **Bach Flower Remedies** – 43 vials

VF 19 **Australian Bush Flowers** – 43 vials

VF 20 **Western Herbs #1**

Miscellaneous, A-Box - 100 vials

VF 21 **Western Herbs #2**

Brooklime – Crawley – 100 vials

VF 22 **Western Herbs #3**

Crosswort – Horsenettle – 100 vials

VF 23 **Western Herbs #4**

Horseradish – Nikkar Nuts – 100 vials

VF 24 Western Herbs #5

Nutmeg – Silver Weed – 100 vials

VF 25 Western Herbs #6

Simaruba – Sma – 100 vials

VF 26 Oriental Herbs – 67 vials

VF 27 Flower Essences – 100 vials

VF 29 Amino Acids – 23 vials

VF 30 Enzymes – 100 vials

VF 31 Total Allergies – 50 vials

VF 35 Organs – 100 vials

VF 41 Glands/Hormones – 100 vials

VF43 Skin, Hair, Nails & Related Conditions – 100 vials

VF 44 Digestive System & Related Conditions – 100 vials

VF 45 Nervous System & Related Conditions – 100 vials

VF 46 Brain & Related Conditions – 50 vials

VF 47 Heart, Circulatory System

& Related Conditions – 100 vials

VF48 Muscular System & Related Conditions – 100 vials

VF 49 Skeletal System & Related Conditions – 100 vials

VF 50 Respiratory System & Related Conditions – 100 vials

VF 51 Urinary System &Related Conditions – 100 vials

VF 52 Immune/Lymphatic Systems

    & Related Conditions – 100 vials

VF 53 Sensory System & Related Conditions – 100 vials

VF 54 Reproductive System – Male

    & Related Conditions – 50 vials

VF 55 Reproductive System – Female

    & Related Conditions – 50 vials

VF 56 Dental & Related Nosodes – 81 vials

VF 60 Psychological Conditions #1

    Negative – 100 vials

VF 61 Psychological Conditions #2

    Positive – 50 vials

VF 62 Psychological Conditions #3

    Psychosomatic – 29 vials

VF 65 Miasms/Propensi – 50 vials

VF 72 **Pain #1**   *Local (Head)* – 100 vials

VF 73 **Pain #2** *Local (Head #2)* – 100 vials

VF 74 Pain #3 *Local (Back)* – 100 vials

VF 75 Pain #4 *Local (Chest)* – 100 vials

VF 76 Pain #5 *Local (Abdomen, Epigastrium)* – 100 vials

VF77 Pain #6 *Local (Abdomen, continued)* – 100 vials

VF 78 Pain #7 *Local (Extremities)* – 100 vials

VF 79 Pain #8

   Types of Pain #1 – 100 vials

VF 80 Pain #9

   Types of Pain #2 – 100 vials

VF 85 Cleansing Kit – 100 vials

VF 86 Detox Kit – 100 vials

VF 87 Human Diseases #1 – 100 vials

VF 88 Human Diseases #2 – 100 vials

VF 89 Organic Rejuvenation – 100 vials

VF 90 Radio Isotopes – 18 vials

VF 97 Cancer – 150 vials

VF 100 Minerals & Their Compounds – 100 vials

In addition to the above, which are all test vials, we offer treatment vials for each test, and the following test and treatment kits:

- 186 Colour Therapy (Chromotherapy) Waveforms
- 33 Common Insect Pests
- 34 Fertilizers
- 37 Insecticides and Herbicides
- 19 Fungicides
- 23 Plant-Derived Drugs
- 34 Chemicals Used in Agriculture
- 600+ Herbs
- 18 Radio-Active Fallout
- 5000+ Diseases and their Causes)
- 28 Chakras
- 14 Acupuncture Channels and all their Points

For additional information, please contact vibrofusion@gmx.com

Please note that **The Kinesiologies Handbook, Volume 2** is in preparation and will shortly be available.

Appendix B

Useful Kinesiology Links

US: INTERNATIONAL College of Applied Kinesiology –
http://www.icakusa.com

Kinesiology Network – http://www.kinesiology.net

International College of Applied Kinesiology –
http://www.icak.com

Wellness Kinesiology –
http://www.wellnesskinesiology.com/

Kinesiologists United –
http://www.kinesiologistsunited.com/

International College of Professional Kinesiology Practice – http://www.icpkp.com/cg/MainMenu

Health Kinesiology – http://www.subtlenergy.com

Chinese Medicine Meridians Used for New Method Kinesiology – http://www.newmethodkinesiology.com/

VibroFusion – vibrofusion@gmx.com

Applied Kinesiology Center of San Francisco, Inc – http://www.aksf.com

Bio-Test – http://www.bio-test.cnchost.com/sys-tmpl/door/

Holodynamic Kinesiology – http://www.drgustafson.com

Global Kinesiology Directory – http://www.kinesiology.nu/

Specialized Kinesiology – http://DrGCD.com

The International Journal of Applied Kinesiology and Kinesiological Medicine – http://www.kinmed.com/

Kinesiology Forum Discussion Lists – http://www.kines.uiuc.edu/forum/lists.html

Manual Kinesiology and Neurokinesiology – http://www.kinesiology.org/

University of Illinois School of Kinesiology – http://www.uic.edu/ahp/knad/home.html

9626958R00177

Printed in Great Britain
by Amazon.co.uk, Ltd.,
Marston Gate.